Natural Hormone Replacement
for Men and Women

How to Achieve Healthy Aging

For orders other than by individual consumers, WorldLink Medical Publishing offers a discount on the purchase of ten or more books. For further details please write to info@mqrx.com or Director of Book Production at 6965 Union Park Center, Suite 100 Midvale Utah, 84047.

For information on how individual consumers can order, please follow the same procedures above.

Natural Hormone Replacement
for Men and Women

How to Achieve Healthy Aging

Neal Rouzier, M.D. FACEP
and Cherie Constance

WorldLink Medical Publishing
Salt Lake City

The stories in this book are reflections of experiences by the author. Patient's names and personal information have been changed to protect their privacy. The recommendations, procedures, and opinions in this book are those solely of the author and are not meant to replace the services of a trained health professional. All matters regarding your health require medical supervision. If you have any preexisting conditions, you should consult with a doctor before practicing any of the procedures within these pages. Neither the author nor the publisher will be held liable or responsible for any loss, injury or damage allegedly arising from any information or suggestion in this book.

Copyright © 2001 By MedQuest Pharmacy.

All rights reserved. No portion of this book may be reproduced in any manner, mechanical or electronic, without written permission from the publisher, except for brief portions, which may be quoted in articles or reviews.

Printed and bound in the United States.

WorldLink Medical Publishing
801-566-5350

Library of Congress Cataloging-in-Publication Data
ISBN 0-9710007-1-9

Book design by Rebecca Findlay

Acknowledgements

To my wife, Carolyn, my personal safety net, who makes the clinics and my endeavors in this field a reality.

To Jacque Bray, whose support and generosity brought this book out of the woodwork.

To Helen Jacot who believed in the power of this book and spent many an hour editing it.

To Rachel Muir for research contributions

To my patients, the true examples of healthy aging, who brought life and personality to this book.

To research teams across the board, who bring credence and significance to the field of preventive and longevity medicine.

But most of all, I dedicate this book to the many doctors who refuse to explore the medical field outside their box. I write this book specifically for you and your patients in hopes that this book will be a catalyst for change, and that patients everywhere will receive the type of preventive therapy worthy of being called patient care.

CONTENTS

Acknowledgments

Forward: Dr. Douglas Dedo   pg - 1

Introduction: My Story of Healthy Aging   pg - 5

DHEA: The Age Gauge   pg - 17

Pregnenolone: Opening your Aging Mind   pg - 41

Melatonin: The Aging Loophole   pg - 49

Estrogen: The Genesis of Hormone Replacement   pg - 63

Progesterone: Estrogen's Natural Side-Kick   pg - 89

Testosterone: Revitalize Every Aspect of Your Life   pg - 107

Testosterone: The Female Side of the Story   pg - 143

Rethinking the Thyroid   pg - 153

HGH: The Ultimate Healing Hormone   pg - 181

Talking the Talk your Doctors Understand   pg - 209

Epilogue: Making the Choice for Longevity   pg - 225

Bibliography   pg - 231

FORWARD

> *...our hormones keep us healthy and when restored to optimal ranges, they keep us energetic and youthful...*
> —Dr. Neal Rouzier

The fountain of youth, that magical elusive spring that Ponce de Leon searched for as an elixir for the aging process, may be closer than we think. Dr. Neal Rouzier has written his answer for the vagaries of aging by sharing with us his story and how it forced him to expand his vision from mainstream medicine to what physicians like to call "alternative medicine." As I write this forward I am torn between writing it from the perspective of a facial cosmetic surgeon, a physician who treats patients with natural, total hormone replacement, or as a patient myself. Just as Dr. Rouzier began his intellectual pursuit of studying the many benefits of natural hormone replacement therapy when he reached his early forties, I too kept my eyes out for the benefits of HGH. I had decided that when I felt life escaping me I would start my own hormone replacement program. Unfortunately, it was illegal for any physician to prescribe HGH unless one was a pediatric endocrinologist. (This despite scientific articles substantiating the efficacy and safety of this hormone.) The major breakthrough that took HGH off the black market was the FDA's approval to prescribe it when blood tests confirmed low levels. Just as estrogen, thyroid and other hormones are replaced, HGH became a part of this important therapeutic program.

In 1997, I began a natural, total hormone replacement program. My energy was declining as my middle age symptoms were increasing. I felt as if my intellectual and sexual function had bottomed out and I was looking at this as being the "standard" of living for the next 22 years, supposing I would die when my father died at 76.

Just as Dr. Rouzier studied the peer review journals for proof behind HRT, I, too voraciously studied everything I could get my hands on to learn more about this program and the aging process. In <u>Natural Hormone Replacement for Men and Women: How to Achieve Healthy Aging</u>, Dr. Rouzier makes it easy for the interested patient to read and understand the effects of each hormone on the aging process and the benefits from their optimal replacement.

Furthermore, Dr.Rouzier does not quote "junk science" but has an incredible bibliography of peer-reviewed journals that would satisfy any professor at a medical school or doctor looking to educate himself. In fact, I would strongly encourage patients to read this book, educate themselves about their choice in the aging process, and then ask their doctor to read it.

I can attest to the kind of difference it has made in my own life. After two months on the program I had lost my gut, my energy levels were back to normal and sexually I was quite pleased. Interestingly, my patients began to comment on my skin and the fact that I seemed to stop aging, which would naturally lead us into a discussion on HRT. Needless to say, my patients also wanted to feel and look better. They too were frustrated by being told "it's the aging process and that they would just have to learn to live with it". So, I began to incorporate longevity medicine in my own practice and many of the testimonies in this book could have come from any number of my own patients.

I personally have found that longevity and preventive medicine is a natural extension of cosmetic surgery. Patients find that they can surgically reverse the effects of gravity and aging through face lifts, eye lifts, etc. and liposuction can reduce the middle age spread and love handles. Yet these procedures can not halt our internal aging process nor make us feel better! I have found that when I prescribe HRT to a patient before surgery, they heal faster and feel better postoperatively. If the patient continues the natural hormone supplements post operatively, I have noticed that two wonderful things happen. First, they will probably never need a second tuck-up or facelift. Second, they will begin to feel good with increased energy, libido, skin texture, muscle-to-fat distribution, and better intellectual function. Most importantly, I give my surgical patients a choice in how they age after the cosmetic surgery!

For those who are interested in an increased quality of life, I ask them to read <u>Natural Hormone Replacement for Men and Women</u>. It answers their questions and makes my job of communicating with their internist much easier (especially if their *doctor* reads the book).

As I have lectured on how to incorporate natural, total hormone replacement therapy into a surgical practice, I conclude with the following to my fellow facial and cosmetic surgeons: It is not IF you will incorporate HRT in your practice but WHEN, because as you age you will demand it for yourself and subsequently for your patients.

Douglas Dedo, M.D.
Palm Beach Gardens, FL.

Introduction:
My Story of Healthy Aging

The reasons for some animals being long-lived and others short-lived, and in a word, causes of the length and brevity of life calls for investigation.
—Aristotle, "The Longevity and Shortness of Life"

Throughout this book I will tell you other people's stories of rejuvenation, but as a reader, it is only fair for you to understand how my own restoration came about. Therefore, I would like to tell you my own story and how hormones have made my aging a healthy and scarcely noticeable one.

Before I became an impassioned believer of natural hormone replacement therapy, I had a firm seat in the conventional medicine camp. I followed the orthodox beliefs of conservative medicine and by doing this I assumed I was serving the common good of man. In the emergency room, I treated situations to the best of my ability, even some that were far from being treatable. I saw too many people with one foot in the grave and the other quickly on its way in the same direction. I simply treated the disease rather than the patient and that was considered the charge of a "good" doctor. I knew how to treat a cardiac arrest or a stroke, yet I had no idea how to prevent these events from happening. Preventive medicine seemed an ideal rather than a reality—little did I know, I had a lot to learn.

My introduction into longevity medicine was basically spurred by selfishness. I just turned forty-three and had started noticing aging's effects creeping into my daily activities. I felt lethargic and my body began to show how I felt. I gained weight, my skin and hair texture lost its healthy glow, and I didn't feel like continuing my disciplined exercise regimen. If I wanted to exercise, I couldn't anyway because I had too much joint pain. Even my passion for racing cars began to wane, and this new reality check, that I was getting old, threw me for a loop. In truth, anxiety hit and I spiraled down into that mid-life crises everyone jokes about. I wasn't laughing. So, instead of giving into aging, I started investigating other, more complex and considered "out there" views of aging. I found a lot of bogus products and programs claiming they had the magic to achieve the restoration of youth, along with a lot of really bad science. I found marketing agents focused on the vulnerable and hopeful who sought out to reverse age-related diseases and physical deterioration. I was frustrated with all the deceptive devices promising the fountain of youth, yet only delivering common amino acids, herbs, and natural substances that have little anti-aging potency and effect.

The Moment of Youth

Among all these silly notions of youth, I stumbled upon natural hormone replacement therapy. This treatment had clinical back-up from peer-reviewed journals and it was gaining respectability and notoriety with each passing month. It not only appeared to work, but it went above and beyond the effects doctors and scientists ever dreamed of expecting. After much investigation and consideration, I sought out a doctor who practiced this kind of therapy, and about a year later began treating my own patients with the powerful benefits of hormone replacement therapy.

I went from a tired, aging man to a vigorous entrepreneur of natural hormone replacement therapy. My workload, which was flagging before, picked up the pace. I had endless energy. I could go to the gym for several hours again, take on ten to fifteen patient cases a day, work on my car, and my wife liked me much, much better after three months of treatment than the whole year prior to the therapy. It was a kind of "born-again" experience, except the source of my redemption was bio identical hormones. I felt like I had stumbled upon the answer to aging and I saw that preventive medicine was truly what the term "patient care" was all about.

With this discovery, I was forced to go through a revolution of thinking about medicine and aging. No longer did I regard it as the human condition, an inevitable lot in life of progressive deterioration, but rather something that could be altered and controlled. I joined the ranks of the minority that treats aging as a disease, and accordingly seeks methods to prevent it. What an awesome notion—we can now take measures to hinder the symptoms of growing older. This was something that the whole world needed to know. With hormone replacement therapy, I felt better and functioned better, yet beyond this I was protecting myself from the deterioration of neurological, cardiovascular, musculoskeletal systems that result in what we call the normalcy of aging.

Supply and Demand

I think it might be possible to modulate the key hormones growth hormone, thyroid hormone, insulin growth factor, and if we can modulate those in a healthy range—maintain our health but toward a level that can permit us to slow aging—I think it's possible to do it.
—Marc Tatar (Longevity Scientist at Brown University).

Humans strive, in spite of the daily examples of aging, to live to a ripe old age. Why is this? I've seen the pattern of older people over the years of practice—bent over, frail, and suffering from age-related declines. This fate is unappealing and nerve-wracking to me, yet I watch what I eat, exercise, and have plans to live well beyond the normal life expectancy. Perhaps this is a facet of the human instinct, something like survival of the fittest. But survival does not necessarily mean a first-rate quality of life. So, the question isn't whether I want to live a long life, but whether I want to ambitiously live a long life of energy and well-being?

I believe the saddest, most deceptive bit of information taught to us as we get older is that what we're experiencing (the cognitive, physical, and emotional declines) are "normal." We're supposed to fall prey to osteoporosis, heart disease, Alzheimer's, and/or cancer, that no one lives forever, and more importantly, no one lives healthy and happily ever after. As a doctor and a patient, I find this kind of apathy frustrating. Yet, I'm excited to say that there is a silver lining, and as I delved into the genre of longevity medicine, I found that major, esteemed medical institutions felt the same way I did and were researching hormones and their anti-aging benefits. Hormones, it seemed, were the key to a longer, more fruitful longevity.

Since the endocrine system, composed of glands that produce and send hormones to various areas of the body, regulates various essential functions of the human body, like temperature, reproduction, growth, aging, and immune system, it stands to reason that it should be science's primary focus as the hub of longevity. And so it is. Science is unraveling the aging code by analyzing each hormone's action and reaction. We are seeing that hormones, at optimal levels, keep the body in a state of homeostasis. If hormones are at healthy levels—the human body is healthy. This ideal functioning of the body can change with many different alterations to the body. The amount of sleep, the kind of diet, and regular exercise influences the levels of our essential hormones. I'm sure you've also realized that the body's homeostasis also declines as we get older. Our physical, emotional, and mental deterioration is a direct reflection of the state of our hormones. Their declining levels influence the rise of disease and complications we associate with age. A change in diet and lifestyle will not delay their decline; rather the decline seems almost preprogrammed. Instead, the best way to alter their decline is through supplementation.

Oddly enough, this desire for youth into age has created a rift in the medical and ethics community. Who are we to mess with Mother Nature, and the ultimate plan of human history for growing older? Who are we to doctor-up the natural sequence of human life—we are born, we get older, we deteriorate, we die—is this not normal? They will contend that this kind of medicine is cosmetic and fueled more by narcissism than by the desire to live longer and better than previous ancestors. You will see, that through this book, I will contest the definition of "normal." I will argue that the conservative doctors and the ethicists do more harm than good and that anti-aging, or more correctly termed, "longevity" or "preventive" medicine, is about more than just vanity, it's about health and a satisfactory quality of life.

Even in light of the criticism, there is a large demand among many people who are contemplating their demise, and seek to find the aging loophole. Forward thinking doctors, like myself, have opened themselves up to the distinct possibility of being the supply to that demand with the clinically proven benefits of natural hormone replacement therapy.

Hormones: The Magic Bullet Program for Aging

Before you delve into the in-depth clinical and applicable descriptions of the powerful hormones, I want to give you a brief taste of the sweet possibilities they can offer an aging body. This overview will only whet your appetite as you begin your own quest for youth and health. You live in an era when aging can be reversed and youth restored. Science and medicine have offered you this opportune moment; I entreat you to seize it.

DHEA: As of late, DHEA, the most abundant hormone in the human body, has become a kind of celebrity of the hormone regimen. Varying opinions either boost its reputation as a multifunctional, age-defying hormone or decry its status, saying it's more hype than substantiation. DHEA has been found to affect the body not only in its own right, but also by way of conversion into testosterone, estrogen, or progesterone. Clinical studies have revealed that DHEA has a profound effect on the immune system, sex drive, metabolism, and one's emotional stability. Its effect on the immune system via regulation of stress hormones and by its function as a powerful antioxidant illustrates one of its age-resisting capabilities. Other health-related benefits include its ability to alter cognitive decline, help the body cope with stress, and exert a healthy influence over the heart by way of cholesterol modulation. Unfortunately, these benefits reverse when its levels decline with age. Whether you believe its supporters or critics, proven studies keep it in the news and in the interest of people who want to remain healthy in their later years. Yet, as a quick side note, even the FDA has also shown signs of approval for DHEA in its use to treat painful diseases like lupus and connective tissue disease.

Pregnenolone: This hormone has been nicknamed the "grandmother hormone," since it is a precursor to DHEA, which is a precursor to testosterone, estrogen, and progesterone. Pregnenolone is most notably recognized for its tremendous memory enhancing properties. Yet, before it was acknowledged for its cognitive boost, pregnenolone was used to treat arthritis. Users reported that they experienced less pain, greater energy and strength, and improved mobility. However, its non-toxic benefits for arthritis were replaced in the 1940's when cortisone was introduced to the market.

It's obvious that as we get older cognitive decline will affect all of us. Certain types of memory fail us, and lack of mental clarity can be one the most frustrating aspects about getting older. Many studies show that pregnenolone may be a powerful adversary against such age-related cognitive diseases as Alzheimer's and may be an important agent against age-associated cognitive declines.

Other possible applications on the horizon for pregnenolone may be in conditions like multiple sclerosis or spinal cord injuries. Studies have shown that pregnenolone may repair the myelin sheath (the fatty layer that protects nerves) and therefore it may be applicable for patients who suffer spinal cord injuries, in the prevention and treatment of paralysis. As with all hormones, pregnenolone's full potential has not yet fully been realized.

Melatonin: This hormone is produced by the pineal gland, the gland some scientists believe to be the source of our body's aging since it controls the activities of virtually every cell in the body. Melatonin regulates the circadian rhythm as well as the deep stages of sleep. Some believe that it is within these deep stages of sleep that the immune system is stimulated. In a January 1997 issue of the *New England Journal of Medicine*, melatonin enjoyed being extolled as a powerful antioxidant, a potential anti-cancer agent, and a perfect candidate to put on the anti-aging roster. Studies using mice have shown that its addition could return 24-month old mice to their more youthful, resilient counterparts.

I believe in light of the hundreds of studies showing that melatonin can scavenge free radicals, fight cancer, induce youthful sleep patterns, and possibly slow the aging process that it's a definite shoe-in for everyone's hormone regimen.

Estrogen: This is the genesis of hormone replacement therapy, and has been prescribed for over 40 years to women suffering the symptoms of menopause, such as hot flashes and moodiness. Yet, because estrogen went above and beyond just staving off the bothersome symptoms of menopause, women opted to continue estrogen therapy and researchers began to explore its other therapeutic realms. Physically speaking, women have seen favorable changes in muscle tone, wrinkles, hair texture, and in their sex lives. Medically speaking, study after study illustrates that estrogen should not be used merely as a treatment of a phase, like menopause, but rather as a lifelong therapy for the determent of such age-related diseases as osteoporosis, Alzheimer's, cardiovascular disease, and depression. Because of the longevity of replacement of estrogen, its beneficial claims are convincing and grounded.

With estrogen therapy, it's not whether or not you should be supplementing your body with it, but rather what *kind* of estrogen you should be using. The estrogen chapter will open your eyes to a new concept of "natural" hormone replacement. Compounding pharmacies now have the capability to formulate and dispense bio identical hormones, or hormones that match exactly the hormones your body naturally produces. It does not make sense to replace your body's hormones with anything but the exact replica of the hormone it's going without. As you read more, you'll understand why.

Progesterone: Another female hormone that works synergistically with estrogen is progesterone. This hormone is commonly overlooked. However, when it is used, it's not for its therapeutic purposes, but rather for its ability to eliminate estrogen's ability to stimulate uterine cancer. Using progesterone for this alone is going about hormone replacement backwards. Progesterone should be looked at as a life-long partner of estrogen or as the balancing ying for yang. An example of this is that progesterone stimulates bone growth, while estrogen halts bone loss. Too many women who have had hysterectomies are not prescribed progesterone, and therefore lack the general make-up of what made them strong and complete in their more youthful years. Natural progesterone works with estrogen by keeping the prevalent diseases of age, like osteoporosis, heart disease, and depression at bay. On its own, it has a mild tranquilizing effect and enhances an overall sense of well being. Studies have shown that it's truly a feel-good hormone.

Testosterone: Although testosterone is the primary male hormone, women also benefit from its supplementation. Levels of testosterone decline in both men and women and as a result, both gain visceral fat, experience a loss in energy, undergo mood swings, and hopelessly watch as their libido goes out the door. At optimal levels testosterone increases bone density and bone formation, enhances energy and sex drive, decreases body fat, increases muscle strength and formation, lowers blood pressure, and modulates the levels of LDL and HDL. Women may not know this, but testosterone is the hormone that keeps their skin soft and supple. Testosterone supplementation is more cost efficient and is an emotionally effective tool in curbing the behavior euphemistically termed "the midlife crises". And to go against the common grain of practice and medical thought, testosterone keeps the prostate healthy. It's a hormone both men and women should not venture into their fifties without.

Thyroid: This metabolic hormone secreted by the thyroid gland regulates temperature, metabolism, and cerebral function, which in turn generates energy and warmth. At optimal levels it breaks down fat, resulting in weight loss, and also lowers cholesterol. The thyroid wards off heart disease and cerebral impairment; however, with age, thyroid levels drop as well. Insufficient thyroid levels result in fatigue, slowness in speech and action, depression, and susceptibility to colds and infection. Perceptible changes include thinning hair and brittle nails. Many of these characteristics sound suspiciously like symptoms of getting on in years. And so they are, yet, they don't have to be. You don't have to be depressed or slow down. The supplementation of a natural thyroid, as opposed to something like Synthroid, can alter what is termed as "normal" aging. Hallmark studies have shown that even when the blood tests show that the patient has normal thyroid levels, supplementing a natural source of thyroid works wonders on energy production in the test subjects. Because of this, I consider the thyroid one of the most misunderstood and underused hormones of the entire replacement program. The thyroid chapter in this book will go against the grain of current conservative medicine, which is, "don't treat a problem if there isn't one." I believe in treating the potential problem so later on there doesn't have to be a problem to treat. This is the key to preventive medicine.

Human Growth Hormone: With the *New England Journal of Medicine*'s publication of the Rudman study, this hormone has made the biggest ripple in the medical community. Growth hormone is the most abundant hormone produced by the pituitary gland and after the age of thirty, it declines at a rate of 14 percent per decade. Studies like that of Rudman's have shown that the supplementation of human growth hormone positively changes body composition by decreasing body fat, while increasing lean body mass; increases bone mass; improves cardiac function and exercise ability; enhances skin texture; and helps to heal wounds faster. This hormone shows rapid results and promises rejuvenation from the inside out—in fact, so much so that Stanford University medical researchers concluded, "It is possible that physiologic HGH replacement might reverse or prevent the inevitable sequela of aging." Because of this, many manufacturers have used the human growth hormone name and corresponding studies to support their invalidated, cheap imitations, i.e., secretagogues (we'll talk in depth about these later in the HGH chapter). I advise you to be wary of these products that espouse a plethora of results without performing the promise.

Natural hormones (described above) are pure pharmaceutical, bio identical (human identical)hormones that are either derived from plants or synthetically manufactured. In this book, I will refer to "synthetic" hormones as the hormones with the side effects. The words natural and synthetic, therefore, get confusing. So, before we go on, I want to clear up my definition of the two words. In this book, when I refer to "synthetic", I mean the chemically altered hormones, like

Provera or Premarin. These hormones do not match the hormones the body makes naturally. "Natural" hormones are an end product, whether naturally or synthetically created, that is identical to the hormones found *naturally* in the body.

A Quick Word of Advice

You may be on hormones now. If you're a woman you may already take a form of estrogen and/or progesterone, but I recommend you to be careful with the types of hormones you supplement your body with. Many women and men are given the synthetic, or altered versions of the natural hormones their bodies produced prior to their age-related drop. It is important to understand the difference in semantics and make-up of the two types of hormones before you venture into the rest of the book.

The drug industry is a huge moneymaking giant. If all else economically fails, I believe pharmaceutical companies will thrive because it is your health, or rather I should say your illness, that they're banking on. These companies entice and educate your doctors in how to treat *your* ailments, and they have the money and marketing expertise to present graphs and studies to "clinically" promote their products. This is why women have been using Premarin and Provera for thirty or forty years now, and why doctors continue to prescribe them, in spite of patient complaints. Because Premarin is comprised of horse urine-derived estrogens, it doesn't take a rocket scientist to comprehend that the human, female body should be supplemented with something that replicates what it normally creates. Provera, a synthetic progesterone, is so molecularly altered that it doesn't fit the receptor sites in the body tissues. In fact, the common side effects of progestin or Provera in the PDR make it sound more like torture than therapy.

This kind of "medicine" may seem as backwards to you as it does to me, but the fact remains: pharmaceutics are money, and natural hormones are not money making products. Natural, bio identical hormones are created in a laboratory to exactly match the hormones your body produces, therefore they cannot be patented—no patent means no financial incentive. This, sadly, is bad science and bad medicine. Synthetic estrogen, progesterone, thyroid, and testosterone are developed to fit the human body as close as possible yet, because of that slight difference can still be unhealthy. They can cause liver problems, edema, and depression. Throughout this book, I will dispel the myths behind these types of hormones and unravel the mysteries behind the natural hormones our bodies make when we are young, and the natural hormones to supplement your body with now that you are older. Cellular receptor sites are best stimulated by bio identical hormones. It's the simple act of deductive reasoning, and this is why it is so hard for me to believe that this is not considered logical or commonplace medicine—after you read this book, I'm positive you'll feel the same way.

What You're Up Against

I should warn you. I should tell you that adding this therapy to your daily upkeep may prove to be harder than you think. I can guarantee that you will most certainly run into criticism from your internist, and perhaps from family and friends. I know that I have had my fair share of arguments with internists, endocrinologists, cardiologists—you name the college of physicians, and I'm sure I've had to explain the method behind what they believe is madness. Ironically, peer-reviewed journals in every specialty of medicine will back me up. I can show cardiologists that testosterone and growth hormone are good for the heart. I can show internists that thyroid insufficiency is not always uncovered by TSH tests and that thyroid even helps what is considered a "healthy" patient. Everything I speak of in this book is not without sufficient backing. And to the doctors that look down their noses with disgust, I only ask them to read their own journals for the information I extol. Interestingly enough, the justification that these hormones will help you live and feel better is not explanation enough for their use. If this reason is not good enough, I honestly don't know what is.

The idea of perpetuated health throughout life may seem too good to be true, and I urge every skeptic who feels this way to continue reading. This book is not opinion based, nor is it a lot of fluff without foundation. Each hormone I discuss and its application to longevity medicine is well grounded with a large amount of clinical backing. So, I advise you to read on and educate yourself in this arena. I can guarantee you this information will help you through the revolution of medicine that is on the cusp of breaking into mainstream treatment, not only for its feel-good benefits, but also because of the tremendous health benefits.

DHEA:
The Age Gauge

People tell me I look better and I know that I feel better. It is like a new lease on life. My doctor can't believe it.
—James, 49

My energy level is unbelievable. I feel as I did when I was thirty.
—Amanda, 56

    I've seen countless patients over the years in emergency situations, and I've seen patients in normal situations where aches and pains are discussed quietly in my office. I've saved lives when hearts have stopped and I've saved lives only when the *potential* of heart failure lurked in the future. All in all, as hard as it is to believe, it is a rarity to receive a thank-you in an emergency setting. Yet, when the quality of a patient's life has been radically improved with hormone replacement therapy, I've received not only thank-yous, but also hugs, heart-felt cards on the holidays, and long-lasting friendships. I suppose the medical practice I'm in is a sort of life-revival, a breathing life back into living, and it's truly extraordinary to watch someone learn to laugh and enjoy the experience of life again. The message I would like to communicate to you, as you read about the all-important subject of aging, is that it doesn't have to be the downward spiral you have witnessed your parents and grandparents fall victim to, but rather an era to look forward to as something you've worked hard to enjoy. The transformations have been truly remarkable, as I have watched old patients become "renewed" patients, and complaints have transformed into testimonials of revived youth and energy. Hormone replacement therapy may not be a cure for dying but I believe, as do many of my colleagues, that it makes life longer, exciting, and much more fulfilling.

We've heard the quintessential stories of patients on the brink of physical and emotional meltdown who, with the help of hormone replacement therapy, have experienced a burst of energy and well-being that is nothing short of a miracle. I understand that these stories can make anyone wary because of their too-good-to-be-true nature, but I've actually seen real life examples and am a living product of what HRT can truly do. I remember particularly a 52 year-old woman—we'll call her "Susan"—who came to me already supplementing with progesterone and estrogen but still complaining of general malaise, accompanied with weakness and muscle pain. Her doctor performed every blood test and dismissed her symptoms as being produced from an overactive imagination, and in turn prescribed her an entourage of antidepressants. This new diet of mood stabilizers neither enhanced her mood, nor caused any sort of relief from the physical pain she experienced day after day. Seeing that "conventional" treatments were not offering Susan relief, a friend referred her to me. After reviewing her blood tests, I prescribed her testosterone, DHEA, and thyroid. With this new regimen, Susan immediately noticed she was no longer fatigued, and her joints and muscles no longer ached. She let me know that her children and husband also perceived a noticeable difference. Her husband was grateful for her renewed interest in their love life, and her children remarked that it felt like the windows were opened and the air had again become light within their home. She felt as young and vibrant as she did before menopause. It's stories like these that reinforce my desire to encourage and take part in studies focused on the human use of natural hormones. It's obvious that every hormone is involved in a complex drama that plays out inside our bodies, and that every hormone is not involved in its own separate monologue but rather all hormones perform with each other, taking cues and signals whether to act or react. In this book, I plan to take each hormone and thoroughly explain its multiple functions so that anyone interested in hormone replacement therapy will understand the pros and cons, and will be able to make a judicious and intelligent decision whether to seek out a physician who is equipped with the know-how and passion for longevity and preventive medicine. There is no reason to sink into age with a disheartened attitude. Instead, with the proper knowledge and motivation, you can take back the reins on your life and enjoy the time you've been looking forward to since you started your retirement fund.

I've decided to start with DHEA because of its widespread use throughout the body. Nicknamed the "Mother of all Hormones" because of its ability to convert into estrogen and testosterone, it also illustrates its own strength apart from being a precursor. It influences aspects of the immune system, stress's impact on the body, the heart and mind, and various age related diseases that alter the way we live as we get older. DHEA is produced by the adrenal glands (glands above the kidneys), as well as the brain and skin, and was believed, once upon a time, to be a sort of "slacker" hormone. It didn't really act like any of the other hormones and seemed to have no direct purpose. Once it was isolated as the hormone that could convert into estrogen or testosterone, it was then believed to be solely a precursor hormone—there to create but not really serving a purpose of its own. It was not until Dr. Norman Orentreich, in 1984, proved that DHEA declined with age, that scientists stood up and took notice and studies began regarding how DHEA affected age, or its flip side—how age affected DHEA.

Another esteemed researcher, Dr. William Regelson of the Medical College of Virginia believes, as do I, that DHEA is one of the best if not the prime example of a biochemical marker for chronological time. You see, by the time we hit eighty, the zona reticularis of the adrenal gland, where DHEA is made, has atrophied, leaving us with 10-20% of the DHEA levels we once had when we were in our mid-twenties. As with all our vital steroid hormones, such as estrogen and testosterone (which I'll discuss more in depth later on in the book), DHEA takes its own age related plunge. This nosedive influences not only the production of the above stated hormones, which of course reflect our gender health, but also the immune system, the heart, the possibility of cancer, and autoimmune disorders like lupus and rheumatoid arthritis, along with affecting our sex drive, sense of well being, and physical appearance. DHEA, the once believed slacker hormone, is now believed to be a sort of "age gauge," a hormone that seems to dictate the quality and quantity of years in our lives. Countless studies have rendered this hormone, not only the most abundant in the human body, but perhaps also the most significant of the hormones in the preventative process. DHEA is definitely one hormone we should never let slip to low levels. It has been shown to inhibit disease, preserve youth, and maintain health. There are even such cases as lupus or osteoporosis, where the disease's symptoms reverse with the administration of DHEA—I will talk about those later in the chapter. I want to begin with the system in the body that is really the culprit behind the advancement of aging—the immune system.

Laid Up With Colds?

DHEA declines at a rapid pace after we leave the golden twenty-something years, as does the efficiency of our immune system. We find ourselves more susceptible to colds and our medicine cabinets jam-packed with the latest flu remedies. From some vitamin combination to prescription drugs, we're trying our best to beat the odds that life seems to dole out with each passing year. It has only been recently that falling hormonal levels have been studied as a source for an elderly immune system's sluggish response to foreign invaders. Even more exciting is that studies are revealing we can actually rejuvenate an aging immune system and stave off the infections commonly found in the elderly with natural hormone replacement therapy. But before I explain how DHEA jumpstarts the immune system, I feel it necessary to clarify the involved workings of the immune system.

The immune system is comprised of many cells bent on keeping the body free from foreign substances like bacteria, viruses, or fungi. These cells retard the active growth of cancer or other diseases that left to their own devices will seize control of the body with tragic results. The body cannot survive without cells like the T-cells, which locate and eliminate foreign attackers; or natural killer cells, which scan the body for abnormal cell growth, like cancer; suppressor cells, which prevent the body from turning on itself in autoimmune disorder fashion; or most important, follicular dendritic cells, which encompass the immune system's ability to recognize or recall the molecular structure of previous foreign antigens and therefore attack on contact. These are what I call the armed forces of the body. Our defense team shields us from the onslaught of meddling substances, but as we age this alliance becomes idle and clumsy in their response to various pathogens. Our body becomes an open playing field, and our team players are growing older and older, while bacteria, viruses, and fungi gain a stronger footing. Because each cell has a direct purpose and each cell impacts the other's performance, when one cell is not as adept as it used to be, the other cells file suit. As we age, so does our immune system's quick and efficient expertise for filtering out even the weakest of colds

Doctors and scientists refer to the aging of the immune system as immunosenescence. Yet, studies are finding that the "normal" age-related decline in immunocompetence is not inevitable. DHEA has proven itself time and time again to prevent the immune system from becoming idle as we put on the years. With proper supplementation of DHEA, our levels can remain youthful, as will the defense mechanisms of our immune system for years to come. The well respected, *Harvard Health Letter* reported in July of 1994 in an article called, "DHEA Gets Respect," that DHEA added to vaccines helped older mice develop and maintain the same assertive antibodies that young mice normally produce. One of the immunosenescence side effects of getting older is our growing inability to react to vaccines. Our immune cells have aged and therefore they cannot recognize or react to the invader the vaccine is trying to impersonate. Therefore, even when an older person is vaccinated with a flu virus, the cells may not have the ability to understand its chemical make up as foreign, or if they do, they won't be able to recognize it when it shows up down the line. Another study, concerning the same subject, illustrated DHEA's ability to restore the immune system's memory so that influenza once again activated the proper channels of response. The body, as it ages, becomes stubborn in its response to such immunizations as the influenza vaccine. With this in mind, a group of scientists observed that 16 and 24-month year old mice immunized with a live influenza virus followed by DHEA treatment, had a marked increase of resistance to a postvaccination intranasal challenge of the live influenza virus. With the help of DHEA, the antibodies necessary were able to rise to the occasion and react to a virus it recognized.

Not only has it been able to enhance certain vaccinations, but it also enhances the immune system as a whole. A 1993 double-blind crossover study involving eleven postmenopausal women demonstrated that 50mg of DHEA daily enhanced natural killer cell activity, and these results were seen in *all* the women. As I mentioned before, natural killer cells within a young and healthy immune system are on the constant lookout for viruses and cancer.

DHEA has also been known to create a trend of immune system recovery in various studies. In our bodies, as well as the bodies of certain animals, there is a sort of communication network that goes on between all the cells in our bodies. Sometimes there is a need to proliferate and other times a need to hold back. These positive or negative responses are initiated by cytokines, the hormone like messengers that transmit information to other immune cells. As we age, the distribution of information is garbled and an instruction to motivate cells to reproduce may be interpreted as an order to block cell growth or vice versa. As you can imagine, this makes matters rather confusing. Cytokines that can do harm like the IL 6, which motivate cancerous cell growth, osteoporosis, and autoimmune disorders can elevate, while IL 2 cytokines that prompt cells to disarm cancerous growth can plummet.

In a study by Dr.'s Samuel Yen, Khorram and Vu (UCSD School of Medicine, La Jolla, California), immunological effects were measured in 65-year-old men supplemented with 50 mg. per day of DHEA. Yen observed an IGF-1 rise of 18%, natural killer cells (the cells that fight cancer) rose by one third and their ability to ward off cancerous cells increased 30-75%! T-cells and B-cells, which combat bacteria, responded more quickly to foreign attackers and IL-2, the cytokine imperative to immune cell communication, also rose significantly.

Another reputable doctor in the pursuit to unravel the hormone mystery, especially DHEA's effects on the aged body, is Raymond Daynes of the University of Utah School of Medicine. He has spent time observing how the immune system and its many facets buckle under the "weight" of age. He has focused specifically on how the cytokines can either be regulatory factors, growth factors, or death factors and how the immune system's health and youthfulness dictate the path a cytokine will take. As I explained before, age creates lapses in necessary communication between cytokines and other cells. These intervals upset a balanced immune system and an over communication of the cytokines, IL 6, IL 10, and IGF, which result in a deregulation within the immune system as we get older. This deregulation enhances the possibility of cancer significantly.

In a study to prove his ideas on DHEA and the immune system, Dr. Daynes created a sort of DHEA cocktail by adding doses of two to eight milligrams a day to a group of mice's drinking water. The effect of the concoction prevented the normal age related cytokine derangement. More importantly, the mice showed dramatic improvements only twenty-four hours after DHEA supplementation, proving that, unlike other medications, DHEA produced fast results. This is noteworthy since IL 6 normally increases nine fold with the onset of age, yet these mice exhibited within twenty-four hours, levels of IL 6 dropping to 15 % within the desired youthful levels. The other problem IL 10 and IGF cytokines were also restored close to normal levels. Another groundbreaking result of this sixteen-month study showed that twenty-four month old mice, basically at the end of their lifeline, when given DHEA, responded to immunizations with the zeal of young mice. All the above beneficial consequences resulting from the addition of DHEA were independent of the thymus gland, which remained shrunken and useless in producing T-cells. Daynes believes, as do I, that although an aged thymus gland negatively affects the immune system, DHEA produces so many other desirable and positive effects that it very well could override the bad. To me, it seems unwise not to continue studying DHEA for its other possible immune enhancing properties.

As I said at the beginning of the chapter, DHEA prevents deterioration rather than restoring lost organ mass that is associated with certain aspects of aging, such as the weakening of the thymus gland. Therefore, early supplementation of DHEA forestalls the shrinkage of the thymus gland, allowing you to catch immunosenescence before it starts. I believe that prevention is the ultimate key to longevity. There is really only one hormone that has been shown through rigorous studies to halt an already aged thymus gland and we'll talk about melatonin later on in the book.

Study after study confirms that DHEA is a veritable treatment for the aging immune system. It recharges NK cells functionality and suppresses the over production of the multifunctional cytokine, IL-6. Researchers have found that DHEA's regulation of IL-6 may in effect eliminate many age related conditions. DHEA-treated mice have illustrated lower levels of serum amyloid P substance, and lowered titers of tissue-specific autoantibodies than what was seen in untreated aged controls. The way we age depends heavily on how healthy our immune system remains. We effectively have the option to inhibit immunosenescence, and in effect, prevent the aging of our own body. With this in mind, I would like to discuss another fundamental facet of aging—stress.

Stress: The Second Pillar of Age

Stress is such an integrated part of our lives. With each passing year, life seems to get faster and we seem to get slower. We're bombarded with some "glorious moments" and sometimes "should haves." There are also "deadlines" and "close calls." We have moments of brilliance, like job promotions or forty years of marriage and also moments of disparity like stock misfortunes or watching someone we love slip into illness. We take the bitter with the sweet and each one comes with its own mess of stresses (those of you who have worked to obtain forty years of "marital bliss" know it's no small feat). All these stresses multiply over the years and sometimes leave less of a person in their wake. You see, sometimes we can't help but internalize stress. We sometimes make it our lifelong companion without realizing its slow, methodical tearing down of our principle vital organs and bodily systems. Some of us believe stress motivates or is a means to the end result or a goal, and to some extent, I agree, but reaching ultimate success is not worth the sacrifice of your health.

Dr. Regelson and Dr. Khorram, both leading researchers of hormone replacement therapy, believe that although DHEA's influence on the immune system does not directly impact the center of immune function, the thymus gland, it indirectly affects immunity by its relationship with stress hormones, corticosteroids. As DHEA alters the way stress is handled internally, it is reflected on how we handle stress externally. The adrenal gland produces corticosteroids to gear us up for emotional, mental, and physical strenuous activity. It is the stress hormones that offer us the energy for fight or flight. With their help, our blood sugar rises and our heart beat increases; in turn, our energy level soars, therefore supplying us with the zeal to make the deadline, survive marital conflict, or endure that wild adventure we euphemistically refer to as "family vacation." Unfortunately, our bodies are not as efficient as we would like them to be and corticosteroids, if not completely employed, can wreak havoc on the immune system, the heart's health, and even on the brain's ability to process and retain information.

Being an emergency physician, I understand the effects of chronic stress. On top of the high volume activity and apprehension, I'm also surrounded by contagious illnesses. I firmly believe that my supplementation of hormones, like DHEA, have shielded me from many complications that disease and stress combined create. They are truly a deadly duo. But by my participation in a hormone replacement program, I feel like I took the normal life expectancy of an ER doctor and in essence, elongated it. However, had I not started an early regimen of hormone replacement therapy, each passing year, the grueling nights in the ER would turn into more corticosteroids loitering in my bloodstream for a longer duration in time. My T-cells would lack the ability they once had to attack quickly and thoroughly. Not only would my immune system falter, but also my heart, mind, and overall well-being.

We know that DHEA declines with age and we also know that our buoyancy to bounce back after a stressful situation also deteriorates while corticosteroids continue to climb. It's a compelling argument then, to say that the dramatic fall of DHEA and the mass production of corticosteroids are closely related to one another. Dr.'s Vernon Riley and William Regelson tested this argument in 1990 by placing a group of mice in harsh and stressful conditions (placing them on a turntable or dunking them in ice water), and then observed how their thymus gland reacted under such severe situations. The thymus gland weakened, shriveled up, and in some cases died. Again, at the suggestion of Dr. Regelson, the turntable test resumed but the mice were first injected with DHEA. With the addition of DHEA, the outcome was radically different. The thymus gland remained unaltered. The mice experienced the same taxing event as the previous group of mice, yet exhibited no signs of internal damage. They were no worse off than they were prior to the study. Dr. Regelson and Dr. Riley then tried to see whether DHEA could rejuvenate an already involuted thymus gland in older mice. They performed the same study with older mice supplemented with DHEA but found no positive transformation within the aged thymus gland. This is why I call DHEA the true preventative hormone. It can alter age before age has altered a person.

Another study also conducted by Dr. Regelson and the esteemed researcher Mohammed Kalimi also illustrated DHEA's awesome strength in combating stress. They gave mice a large dose of dexamethasone, a hormone disguised as a stress hormone release, causing blood pressure to skyrocket. After the injection, a large majority of the mice died from either heart failure or stroke. But with supplementation of DHEA before the injection of dexamethasone, the mice survived while maintaining normal blood pressure levels. DHEA stopped a stress-induced disease in its tracks. In both studies, DHEA took seemingly deathtrap situations and worked its preventative magic.

Corticosteroids have also been seen to negatively affect the brain. I'm sure you've noticed that stress strains the brain's short-term memory. I remember before I started my own hormone replacement program, when I was under a large amount of stress, my short-term memory faltered. With supplementation of DHEA as well as other hormones, I found that I was better equipped to handle tension more efficiently. It seemed as if my brain had undergone a tune-up. Initial studies have verified this by showing that DHEA has potent anti-glucocorticoid actions on the brain, and can protect hippocampal neurons from glucocorticoid-induced neurotoxicity.

Because of this, I find it ludicrous that DHEA should be scoffed at as a "slacker hormone." The high DHEA/low corticosteroid ratio is really a key to the anti-aging process. I include DHEA in my own hormone replacement regimen because of the fast and hectic life I live. Of course I love my life this way, and as years pile one on top of the other, I feel assured that I control my own rate of aging. There is no doubt in my mind that DHEA makes you feel better, look better, and live longer. It's up to you to choose whether you would like to live, look, and feel healthier into your fifties, sixties, seventies and beyond.

Cancer: The Rooted Disease

And we know nothing about such pain...
—Ellen Bryant Voigt

I remember in med school looking in awe at pictures of the how cancer sprouts and grows. An ulcerated mass extends its malignant tendrils like an unruly rooting system and plows throughout the body as if it were loose dirt. This is a quiet act, for although cancer is ruthless, its violent riot is done peacefully, sometimes without the slightest indication of its presence. Our healthy cells are silently robbed while we surf the Internet, enjoy the first bite of a well cut and cooked steak, or while we take our morning jog before work. While we're living, we're essentially dying, and the whole time, unaware we're hosting a web of cancerous growths.

As I explained before, the immune system has many cells watching for any indication of a cancerous growth. In an ideal situation, our immune system would never have to rush to the rescue. Under normal and desired conditions, our bodies replenish cells as they die, with both young counterparts and what is called "stem cells." Stem cells are immature cells with the ability to mass-produce new tissue. As they get older they must jump certain hurdles to reach full maturity, and as they get closer to full maturity, their potential for generating new tissue tapers off, allowing them to function as mature cells. Sometimes though, a cell's growth becomes stunted or suspended. Instead of going on to healthy adulthood, they form a clump of abnormal, immature cells called a tumor. If the disruption of cell growth happens close enough to cell maturity, the tumor is benign. It actually even resembles a healthy adult cell, and grows slowly without invading other tissues or making a nuisance of itself.

However, if the cessation of growth takes place while the cell is still immature, or when it has the potential to reproduce, the chance of malignancy is eminent. Something genetic, environmental, or chemical has provoked these cells to never "grow-up" and take the responsibilities they were intended to take as mature cells. Instead of worrying about respiration, a cancer cell in the lung is more concerned with production of more cells like itself, creating a gang of cells that cause trouble for the tissue they were intended to support. Their deranged structure also affords them the luxury of immortality. They never die and they always reproduce, defying the laws of nature on every scale. The sad part is that the cancer victim may only find out when symptoms cannot be ignored or a wandering hand discovers an unfamiliar growth. Then it may be too late.

The problem with conservative medicine is that many doctors believe that if you don't have a disease, why treat it, right? This has been the thought process for many years, and in the mean time we are like sitting ducks, waiting for an illness before taking measures to preserve the precious terrain of our bodies. I believe this concept of medicine has only instigated disease. It is rare, except in extreme environmental conditions or predisposed geneticND dispositions, that a child falls prey to cancer. A child or young adult still has hormone levels that amplify the immune system's ability to search the body like a fine-toothed comb for any disturbance, such as bacteria or cancerous growths. Cancer, most times is an age-related disease. And although DHEA is in the beginning stages of study as a method of cancer prevention, it has been shown, in many instances, to be a hormone that can thwart cancer. A Dr. Arthur Swartz of Temple University found that, within cell cultures, supplemental DHEA actually insulated cells from the toxicity of carcinogens. Normally carcinogens, like the kind caused by smoking, mutate cells by fooling with their DNA structure, or deform cells by changing their actual physical appearance, and in the end cause the once healthy cells to die. With the addition of DHEA, these results were diminished significantly.

How does DHEA stop a normally violent and powerful cascade of reactions that exposure to carcinogens, like smoking, normally causes? DHEA halts the course of events in a sneaky and indirect fashion. Instead of going to the source, it inhibits the enzyme glucose-6-phosphate dehydrogenase (G6PDH). This enzyme stimulates the chemical, NADPH, which triggers a tumor to become malignant.

DHEA is the mechanism of anti-initiation and anti-promotion in some cases of carcinogenesis. DHEA essentially stops this disastrous chain of events at the very get-go.

Another interesting study illustrated DHEA's ability to work against a mouse leukemia retrovirus. The researchers observed an infected group of mice and a control group. Both were supplemented with varying doses of DHEA. The uninfected mice administered .06% of DHEA showed an increase in IL-2 (interleukin-2), gamma interferon production, and hepatic (liver) vitamin E levels. In the infected group, the normal induced severe oxidative stress was reduced by DHEA supplementation. It stimulated the production of cytokine IL-2 and IFN-gamma, while suppressing the production of IL-6. Immune dysfunction and increased oxidation were largely prevented by DHEA.

Studies are under way now to see if this could be the end result. Dr. William Regelson reports in his book <u>The Super Hormone Promise</u> of his own tests conducted on cancer patients. Over a two-and-a-half-year period, Dr. Regelson gave high dosages, based on the weight of the patient, ranging from 2800 to 3200 mg daily. (These dosages were based on the state the patients were in, and are not condoned to be used, under any condition, without proper doctor supervision.) The patients reported a rise in energy and a decrease in fatigue from DHEA. Two of the patients suffering from terminal kidney cancer were able to extend their life expectancy beyond two years. During that time, although DHEA could not cure the cancer, its fatal effects were delayed. Regelson related that DHEA yielded the patients a sort of mercy from the pain cancer is rarely without. DHEA gave the patients hope.

Hope is the one sure answer for cancer at our present time. We have made leaps and bounds in the science community, but still have not found any definitive cures for this malicious disease that broods in our bodies while we go about our normal business. Administration of DHEA to laboratory mice has been shown to prevent varied forms of cancer within the breast, lung, colon, liver, skin, and lymphatic tissue. Regelson believed in the hope that DHEA may show the same benefits in humans and to illustrate his confidence, he tested it on patients. To his delight he found gracious results. DHEA did not cure the cancer but it borrowed back a few years from it—to a cancer patient, years are rare jewels. Like any hormone, self-supplementation is never suggested. Because of its ability to convert into testosterone or estrogen, a person with cancer or the potential of cancer should always consult a doctor before purchasing an over-the-counter "cure." Yet even with these prudent warnings, there is a definite positive effect seen in the relationship of DHEA and cancer. It's amazing that our own bodies hold the key and provide the hope, although as we grow older, they need a little outside supplementation of familiar hormones to feel healthy again.

A Hearty Hormone

As our hormones each take their final bows and one by one dwindle and disappear from the stage of our body, our critical organs and bodily systems acquiesce to aging's overpowering dominance and we begin to die. There are the quintessential outside appearances of age, easily recognized by the graying and loss of hair; thinning, wrinkling, and the emergence of age spots in the skin; fingernails becoming brittle and breaking; and an overall bending under what I refer to as the "weight of age." Our blood no longer runs so smoothly through our veins, causing these visual outputs of age to become apparent. Blood is our life source; even the smallest particles in our cells depend on it. When it stops pumping effectively, our entire body feels the effect, from our memory down to our ability to function sexually. The organ most influenced by blood loss is our pacemaker. Coronary heart disease is the leading cause of death in America and we're all at risk of becoming one of its victims.

There are contributing factors to whether or not a person will develop heart disease. In industrial countries, like America, we actually cater to heart-unhealthy lifestyles. We've made bad food easily accessible by creating drive-through windows so you never have to leave your car. We've invented all sorts of gadgets for the sole purpose of promoting idleness. We have remote controls to operate all the electrical appliances (clapping got too hard) in our houses, we use products like "Exercise in a Bottle," so we never have to touch our toes again, and our lives are clogged with a variety of products that are actually ensuring an early retirement to the grave. Life may seem easier for the time being, but as our hormones drop, along with all our youthful support systems, this indolent life style plays catch-up. Our bodies are no longer equipped to handle the stress of the "good life." By eliminating life's small "inconveniences," we have shackled ourselves to our own self-assured fate. But, if we can influence our destiny in a negative way, then it seems viable that we can manipulate our fate positively. We can stop our heart from also jumping on the aging bandwagon.

I want to pause here for a moment before I explain how the heart struggles with age. I want you to understand its incredible precision while it is in its healthy form. There are four chambers divided into upper atria and lower ventricles and also divided into left and right. The atria is basically the receiving chambers, while the ventricles are the pumping chambers. Each side of the heart has a different role in how the blood is recycled. The right side of the heart receives "used" blood returning from the tissues and drives it through the lungs to aerate it, then the left side admits the newly oxygenated blood and pumps it throughout the rest of the body. The actual pumping action has amazed doctors and scientists for years because of its powerful force. The left ventricle has the thickest and strongest wall of the four chambers, allowing it to propel about 2 1/3 ounces of blood with one single push (about 14,000 pints a day). The heart never rests.

The most common form of heart disease is atherosclerosis, which takes place when the arteries become narrowed and jammed. A thick, yellowish substance called plaque adheres to the inner lining of the arteries, causing the heart's alleyways to become clogged. This plaque is mostly comprised of low-density lipoproteins (bad cholesterol) and triglycerides along with other debris carried in by the blood. As the plaque grows, it bands together with neighboring plaque and, in a sense, cements the inner walls into a traffic jam. This roadblock causes the body's pacemaker to go into overdrive, working harder as its blood supply is reduced. The heart is essentially strangled, and with its death, the rest of the organs go into shock and also die.

The odds to develop heart disease skyrocket after we hit the ominous fifty-year mark. I believe it all relates to the decline in our most important hormones. This is DHEA's cue.

Women are less susceptible to heart disease at the time men are worried about or suffering from it. It is only after menopause that women catch up to their spouses. Yet, low levels of DHEA seem to be more of an indication for men as to whether or not they will be forced to brave the world with a sickened heart. An early study in 1986, in *The New England Journal of Medicine*, conducted by Elizabeth Barratt-Connor at the University of California, measured the DHEA sulfate levels of 242 men over a twelve-year span. The men with higher levels lived longer and were less likely to suffer from heart disease, unlike the men with low levels who seemed predestined for heart problems.

Another study followed 1,709 men from 1987-1989, when baselines were ascertained through blood tests, through 1995-1997, when again blood tests were gathered and assessed. The men with the lowest serum DHEA at baseline recordings were shown to significantly incur ischemic heart disease. This was still the case when other risk factors for heart disease were taken into account, like obesity, smoking, and diabetes. These results clearly indicated that DHEA serum levels were warning signs for future heart disease problems.

So how does DHEA sustain a healthy heart and interfere with the natural process of aging? DHEA, when maintained at youthful levels, keeps bodily systems working in sync with one another. Without DHEA, certain factors work against the body. Common allies to the body and mind's wellbeing, like stress hormones (as we discussed before), insulin, and platelets, turn against us, and where they once served to ensure the body's youth and vitality, now cause a sort of chaos that escalates into aging.

Insulin, a necessary hormone secreted by the pancreas is needed by everyone for energy storage and protein synthesis. Insulin is essential to promote synthesis and storage of glucose (for short term energy) and fat (for long term energy). Insulin also stimulates the formation of proteins (the body's building blocks) from amino acids. But as I said before, age drops the levels of some hormones while increasing the levels of others. In this case, there is a rise in insulin levels, which is a product of age, while DHEA levels decrease. This teeter-totter effect can cause such problems as Type II diabetes.

As I said before, diabetes is a sure path to heart disease. As we get older some of us will develop Type II Diabetes, or "adult onset diabetes," the most common form of diabetes. The most obvious reasons that factor in evolvement of this type of disease are obesity and lack of exercise. In this kind of diabetes, the body is not dependant on insulin. This is also called "insulin resistance," and left unencumbered can cause high blood pressure, high cholesterol, kidney failure, and obesity. Insulin moves glucose from the bloodstream to the inside of body cells. This glucose, or sugar, then becomes an important source of energy for the cells of the body. Because insulin receptor sites on target cells in skeletal muscles and on the liver decline in sensitivity, the surplus of glucose in the bloodstream sends our whole system off kilter. The high glucose levels then damage blood vessels, causing major circulatory problems in the extremities, like the legs and arms.

As far as blood vessels are concerned, type II diabetes can do either of two things: cause unwanted or untimely spasms, blocking blood from flowing to the heart, or cause the blood vessels to stiffen, interfering with the pumping of blood and possibly causing damage to the vessel itself. The effects of type II diabetes has also been shown to inhibit the production of capillaries, small blood vessels. This repression causes a sort of "nerve wilting" in the arms and legs. The complications of diabetes, in a sense, speeds up the process of aging.

So how does DHEA fit in this? A large amount of evidence indicates that DHEA may play a defining role in decreasing the chance of cardiovascular disease. In a thirty day, double blind, placebo controlled 1995 study, Jakubowicz, Beer, and Rengifo reported the results of supplementing twenty-two men aged fifty-seven years with 100 mg of DHEA. Serum insulin levels dropped from 35.3 to 25.8 microgram/ml and serum glucose dropped from 93.4 to 88.9 mg/ml. In the placebo group the serum levels in both glucose or insulin showed no remarkable change.

As I have already mentioned, women are relatively safe from heart disease prior to menopause, but after the change of life, and all hormones decrease, the risk becomes quite serious. Several studies have testified to DHEA's powerful ability to curb insulin resistance in women. Two studies in 1995 by opposite teams of researchers showed how DHEA at 50 mg a day quelled an insulin dominance. P. Casson and colleagues found that "T-lymphocyte insulin binding and degradation increased with DHEA. Enhancement in T-lymphocyte insulin binding and degradation is a previously defined marker of insulin sensitivity."

Diabetes may be a common household name, but there is nothing commonplace about it. As I stated before, obesity plays a large role in the onset of adult diabetes. Sometimes a proper diet and exercise regimen will eliminate these symptoms and of course I always advocate a healthy maintenance of body and mind but in some cases it's not enough. DHEA has been proven, at optimal levels, to arrest insulin production to lower, more normal levels.

A study conducted by Les Coleman PH.D. of the Jackson Laboratories in Bar Harbor, Maine in 1983, supplemented DHEA to a breed of mice predisposed to diabetes. The results spoke for themselves. The mice neither developed diabetes nor became obese. In humans, as J.E. Nestlor reported, DHEA can be raised again by using medication that lowers insulin and restores DHEA levels in old men back to what they were in their youth. Insulin stops the synthesis of DHEA and accelerates its breakdown. If we can maintain our levels of DHEA at optimal levels, we'll keep the teeter-totter effect on our side. There is no reason why diabetes should become a household name in your home.

DHEA has also been shown to have some anti-obesity functions. Studies in obese animals have shown that supplemented with DHEA, they have significant weight loss compared to placebo treated animals. A specific study of spontaneously obese dogs illustrated that with the supplementation of DHEA the dogs had a significantly greater reduction in fat than the placebo-treated dogs. Not only this, but the DHEA-treated dogs had a 32 percent reduction in total plasma cholesterol (of that percentage, there was 27 percent decrease in high density lipoproteins and a 50 percent decrease in low density lipoprotein). The importance of this study is that both groups of dogs were put on a caloric restriction plan, yet it was only the dogs supplemented with DHEA who experienced the fastest rate of weight loss and the desirable shift in their lipid metabolism.

Another study along these lines used rats fed high fat diets which resulted in visceral obesity and muscle insulin resistance. The researchers used two groups of rats, one administered with DHEA and the other without. The group fed DHEA along with a high-fat diet was protected against an increase in fat and a decrease in insulin-stimulated muscle uptake. The mice without the beneficial supplementation of DHEA experienced a two-fold greater visceral fat mass and 50 percent lower rate of maximally insulin-stimulated uptake.

These studies were done primarily on animals, yet I have seen the same kinds of effects in my patients. It also gives hope to those who have tried all the diet plans and have been unsuccessful in their pursuit for a healthier lifestyle. DHEA along with a restricted caloric diet did wonders for the dogs, and even without less calories, the mice did not experience weight gain. I believe more studies are in order before the jury is in, but as far as I'm concerned, DHEA is a veritable enemy against age-related fat gain and muscle loss.

Finally, DHEA works as an antioxidant. A recent study in the *Journal of Lipid Research* indicated that DHEA had antiatherogenic effects through its relation to HDL and LDL lipoproteins. In this particular study, researchers observed the presence of DHEA in relation to the changes in HDL and LDL lipoproteins with age. They also monitored the susceptibility of LDL to oxidation with age in the presence of DHEA or vitamin E. Vitamin E was unable to restore the decreased resistance to oxidation in elderly subjects, yet DHEA, an integral part of a balanced LDL and HDL ratio, increased LDL resistance to oxidation in a concentration manner. The researchers hypothesized that DHEA scavenged directly the free radicals produced by the oxidative process.

Age is a formidable enemy of the heart. From insulin resistance, to weight gain, to cholesterol build up, to stress, the heart is overwhelmed by these overachieving enemies. DHEA can be a true protagonist in the story of the heart and an absolute antagonist to the heart's foes. At youthful levels, DHEA keeps insulin in check, is an excellent antioxidant, and buffers the heart against stress. DHEA may be the heart's best medicine. Without it, we may as well be sitting ducks, waiting to be the next statistic.

Adagio For Looking and Feeling Good

Depression affects about 15 percent of our population and a large part of that number happens to fall in the aging population.

There are many things that factor into why our mood takes the plunge. Age robs us of a sense of security, well-being, and self confidence. We begin to falter in areas that, at one time, we felt we had a firm grip on. Some people actually go into a sort of "hiding" after they reach a certain age, because they can't handle watching themselves slow down in a world that suddenly got too fast. Our energy drops and we feel winded doing normal household chores. We see extra pounds piling on our waists and thighs. And then, I suppose to cope, we become complacent. The symptoms of age are matter of fact, we settle into our lives of avoiding mirrors and opting for escalators over stairs. We basically hand over our fate, and wait. And what are we waiting for? Are we biding our time for it to finally be over? I see this resigned face day in and day out, in the check out lines of grocery stores, while I'm stopped at a traffic light, and finally in the hospital, where any left over fight is quelled by tubes and needles. Above all, I believe this kind of apathy to be the true killer. It's what cancer and heart disease truly feed on. This loss of hope and passion for living are the true culprits of aging.

At the beginning of this chapter I told you that I loved my job, and I will tell you again, there is nothing better than listening to an enthused voice over the telephone telling me they have come out of hiding and with the help of hormone replacement therapy, joined the living.

I remember specifically a fifty-five year old banker, "Jake." He had fallen into the rut of resignation. He felt he needed to retire, that he no longer had the drive or passion for job projects. In effect, he wanted to go into hiding. This lack of appetite frightened him. He no longer had the creative juice nor mental sharpness he was once admired for. He forgot important dates, deadlines, and projects. His mind and body began to let him down. Some of his friends had had encouraging experiences with hormone replacement therapy and recognizing his aging complacency, they recommended him to me. I devised a program of HGH, thyroid, testosterone, and DHEA and after a few weeks, he began to notice an obvious turnaround. He reported a renewed energy and vigor for his job. He now thrives under pressure and enjoys beating the odds, all this from a man who almost passed up the only chance to live again.

I've related only partly why our moods suffer. I also want you to understand biologically what happens to the endocrine side of things. The hormones and related organs and glands that create or stimulate hormones comprise our endocrine system. Everything related to our breathing and thinking depends on the proper functioning of our hormones. Our hormone levels go through a series of changes over the years, which directly affect the activity of most cells within the body. Our hormones decrease, and whether age is the culprit behind the decline in our cardinal hormones or whether our declining hormones incite age, it doesn't really matter. The key issue here is that age and decreasing hormones go hand in hand. In this chapter, I've gone into great detail on the certain aspects of age that ravage the body: cancer, heart disease, stroke, and diabetes and how DHEA supplementation can alter these chain-of-events from happening. But now I want to focus on how age influences our emotional and intellectual outlook and how the decline in mood and thinking ability influences how we age and where DHEA supplementation fits into this area of aging.

One of DHEA's most substantial effects is on energy and well-being. I have countless stories of personal experiences and the experiences I've witnessed in my own patients. One of my patients calls it her "pick-me-up pill." She says it was like she could get through a day again without the desire to crawl under her desk and take a quick nap. Beyond the personal patient accounts (which are just as important), there is also a large body of hard, documented proof that DHEA induces a sense of mental and emotional health while promoting stamina. What's interesting about all these reported increases in mood and energy is that they were not what the tests were conducted to prove. They were added bonuses. In a 1995 study at the University of California School of Medicine, thirteen men and seventeen women were administered 50 mg of DHEA for six months. Among other benefits, the men and women also reported a "physical and psychological well-being for men (67%) and women (84%)." They attributed this boost of activity and frame of mind to the DHEA-influenced rise of serum IGF-1 levels and its increased bioavailability to target tissues.

In 1996, a twelve month study using a DHEA cream on fifteen 60-70 year-old women was conducted to determine its anti-osteoporosis and bone-building benefits. Not only were these hypotheses proven, but 80% of women experienced an increase in mood and overall well-being as well as scores for depression and anxiety.

In another more recent 1999 study, M. Bloch et. al. took fifteen patients suffering from midlife dysthymia (minor depression). There was a 60 percent positive response during the DHEA phase and only a 20 percent positive response during the placebo phase. There was a general restoration of joy, energy, and motivation. The lackluster numbness, sadness, and inability to cope with stress, which accompanies age and instigates illness, were stifled by DHEA's influence.

So many of my new patients complain of no longer enjoying life. They see the years stretch out and their eyes glaze over with a general despondency. They have seen doctors, psychiatrists, herbalists, anyone to offer an answer that works. Unfortunately, the usual answer received and the same cure-all, a prescription mood stabilizer that more often than not creates a neurosis rather than curing one. With a total hormone replacement plan, the patient is supplied with a natural product the body is lacking with the onset of age. DHEA offers great relief from many potential side effects of age, with only a small amount of potential side effects from its use.

Where To Start

There are only a few things to consider when taking DHEA. High doses are usually well tolerated although not advised, and few side effects have been reported. Some suffer from moderate acne or hirsutism, but this can be avoided or remedied by lowering the dosage. With hormone replacement therapy, the fundamental component is always replacing the hormones to *optimal* levels. Not just barely enough to get to normal levels nor superseding what is required, but getting the levels back to where they were during youth levels. This kind of therapy rarely induces side effects.

DHEA has been through the research wringer for over forty years. Researchers have not yet uncovered any dangerous setbacks, yet there is still apprehensiveness in its recommended use. As with all of hormone replacement therapy, many researchers feel we should wait for a more definitive answer and therefore become fence sitters. I have seen and been a part of the experimental process in my own right. DHEA has a long list of proven positive effects, and it's obvious that its decline influences many of the age-related diseases and complications we're supposed to live through while they make up their minds whether or not it's appropriate medicine. I have given you the proof, not only in stories, but also in studies—you now can decide if you want to join the fence sitters, or join in on longevity. Think of all the years waiting to be lived.

Pregnenolone:
Opening your Aging Mind

I haven't noticed any ground breaking changes, just a subtle transition of mental clarity. I've also perceived a more optimistic outlook—I mean I actually feel better.
—Jack, 65

When I told my family doctor that I was forgetting more often and that I was not on top of my game anymore, he said it was "normal for my age." For a top business consultant, I have learned to hate that phrase. My doctor now gives me natural hormones, like pregnenolone, and I'm back on top again. I'm proud to say, I'm functioning quite "abnormally for my age."
—Barbara, 59

We've all watched someone in our lives wither under the weight of age. Whether it is a parent, grandparent, or family friend, we have encountered a glimpse of the reality of growing old. We accept this fate as one day being our own and instead of being taught otherwise, our society only instigates the myth that the diseases and symptoms that accompany age are indeed, facts of life. However, hormone replacement therapy offers a scientific approach that can make aging significantly less noticeable to you and your family. We can't literally stop the clock, but we can potentially lengthen life and make it worth living. As you will learn in this book, the true miracle workers behind staying young are the hormones in our body. With their constant maintenance, with proficient and knowledgeable titration of hormone levels from a healthcare practitioner, the aging crisis becomes a past concern. Every hormone plays a part in our youth, and whether these hormones seem familiar in name or practice, their essentialness to the body will become obvious as you continue to read. One of the most innocuous, yet beneficial, players amongst these indispensable hormones is pregnenolone.

After reading the first chapter, you know that DHEA is called the "mother" hormone, since it is a precursor to estrogen and testosterone. Pregnenolone is the precursor to DHEA, which gives it the nickname the "grandmother" hormone, the genesis of steroid hormones. Because pregnenolone is a precursor to the important steroid hormones in our bodies, you can only imagine how with its decline, our bodies suffer the consequences of aging.

Pregnenolone, manufactured from cholesterol, is produced in the brain and the adrenal cortex, the glands above the kidneys. Because of this, scientists have studied it in hopes that it may be the key to the brain's health and longevity. Like DHEA and the other hormones in this book, its levels decline as we age and when we hit our mid-seventies, we have *60 percent* less than we did when we were in our prime. It seems therefore, no coincidence that our mental health deteriorates about the same time we are significantly lacking this all-important neurosteroid.

Although pregnenolone serves the role as a potent precursor to other hormones, alone it works to keep the brain functioning at peak capacity. Its levels are highest in the brain and studies have shown that it enhances many of our mental functions. New and exciting research has also shown that pregnenolone works as a cellular repairer, particularly in the brain and nerve tissue and it protects cerebral function by guarding against neuronal injury. The future is bright for pregnenolone, and as research continues to uncover the many mysteries behind its needed replacement, its reason for use becomes emphatically clear.

Pearls of Wisdom

So far, we've talked a lot about what hormones do for the body—and how a decline in hormone levels causes or contributes to a string of negative symptoms we associate with aging. But as much as we dread the physical decline that accompanies aging, we also worry about decreases in our mental faculties: the loss of short-term and long-term memory, a drop in mental acumen and alertness, even a general lack of interest in living. We don't learn as well, think as rapidly, or remember things like we used to when we were younger.

Progressive memory loss and related cognitive dysfunction have become overwhelming age-related medical and social problems. According to the United States National Institute on Aging, there are four million cases of the form of dementia related to Alzheimer's disease. This, of course, is the worse case scenario of cognitive decline, so just think of the widespread unreported cases of mere mild cognitive impairment. Unfortunately, this number will only grow as we as health care practitioners and patients dismiss it as the universal story of getting older.

This is where pregnenolone steps in. What the other hormones are to the body, pregnenolone is to the brain. In countless studies, pregnenolone has been shown to reverse age-related deficits in spatial memory performance and to have protective effects on memory in different models of amnesia. With its inclusion in your hormone regimen, you can effectively intervene in what history has claimed as normal, and put a halt on cognitive aging.

In the mid-1940's, pregnenolone gained recognition when its memory-enhancing effects were studied in a variety of tests that measured hand-eye coordination, learning, and memory skills. In one, subjects learned how to use a "flight simulator." The researchers discovered that the subjects taking pregnenolone, regardless of their previous flight experience, faired better than those on placebo—mental effects were seen just after taking pregnenolone for two weeks. Their hand-eye coordination improved and their memory of the drills sharpened. Still more studies involving factory workers yielded similar results—both their memory and learning was enhanced.

Unfortunately, after the 1950's, pregnenolone was put on the back burner for what I believe an unfortunate amount of time. Back before it was recognized for its brain boosting benefits, it was used to treat rheumatoid arthritis, and as a form of arthritis therapy it worked rather well. Patients on its therapy demonstrated marked improvement in the degree of pain and swelling of joints that are commonly associated with the disease. Yet, being a hormone and FDA regulated, its production was economically unproductive and pharmaceutical companies turned to more lucrative products, which could be patented such as cortisone, a close cousin to pregnenolone, as a means of therapy for the painful symptoms of rheumatoid arthritis. Pregnenolone it seemed, for the time being, had lost its edge in the medical field.

However, in the 1990's, pregnenolone skirted the patent issues. The Dietary Supplement Act of 1994 stated that any food derivative or extract could be sold without permission from the FDA. Pregnenolone, which is created from cholesterol, is not only viewed as a food derivative but also has no adverse effects, and, therefore, is not under the jurisdiction of the FDA. With what scientists already knew of its potential benefits, interest in pregnenolone soon increased.

Numerous new studies have confirmed pregnenolone's awesome capabilities as a memory enhancer that makes both learning and retaining information easier. Several of these studies have been printed in the esteemed journal, *Proceedings of the National Academy of Sciences,* and in the last few years research on pregnenolone's impact on memory and learning has become an issue of popularity and interest.

A study cited in the January 1992 issue involved a group of male mice supplemented with different hormones and put through "foot-shock active avoidance training." Observations on how well the mice retained information found that pregnenolone was the most potent and resulted in the best retention of information. The researchers concluded that in light of the age-instigated decline of pregnenolone along with the many cholesterol-blockers (remember, pregnenolone is cholesterol derived) prescribed to older people, the supplementation of pregnenolone is of utmost importance for its cognition-enhancing benefits.

Dr. Morley emphatically believed in pregnenolone's necessity for the aging mind. After he researched and observed its benefits in experiments he performed on mice, he related it to an assured therapeutic shoe-in to battle the virtual epidemic of mental decline associated with aging in humans. "It is clearly by far the most potent of the neurosteroids for improving memory by light-years, and it has a much broader memory response than any of the other neurosteroids. This makes it almost an ideal agent for looking at memory and the consequences of the age-related deterioration of memory."

Another study, reported in the November 1995 issue of the same magazine, showed equivalent supportive results. After pregnenolone, DHEA, or corticosterone were injected into the hippocampus of mice who had once been weakly drilled in foot-shock active avoidance training, scientists observed how well they recalled their exercises. Of all the hormones tried, pregnenolone required the lowest doses to achieve the highest memory enhancing ability.

Other studies have shown that pregnenolone not only enhances memory but may also inhibit memory deficits induced by drugs. An August 1996 issue of *Psycopharmacology* reported the effects of mice that were induced with scopolamine and pregnenolone. Scopolamine typically causes learning complications and retention performance deficits in the tasks the mice were continually run through. By adding pregnenolone, the usual scopolamine-induced learning deficiency was blocked, moreover; the addition of pregnenolone actually enhanced their memory capabilities.

Most of my patients, before they came to me, have never heard of the hormone pregnenolone. They of course have heard of the diseases (Alzheimer's and cognitive decline) that result from low pregnenolone levels, but they don't quite understand the cause and effect process. After they have been on pregnenolone and the other hormones that complete the longevity equation, they think and feel better. One patient, in particular, said he felt like the program had unclogged his brain. He didn't feel like he had to sort through memories anymore. These types of comments and personal accounts make being a physician in this field a worthwhile endeavor.

Since it helps with the formation of the myelin sheath (membrane that surrounds and insulates our nerve fibers) over cells, it has been revealed to improve the transmission of nerve impulses, and build bridges of communication between brain cells. Because of this, some doctors and scientists believe it to be one of the most powerful and safe memory enhancers ever.

Pregnenolone was one of the first hormones determined to be both safe and effective. The brain is your ally, your defense against disease and stress. Without pregnenolone, as we age, the brain can go down the same path of decline as the body. You owe it to yourself to stay alert, to keep your memory intact, and to enjoy life as long as possible.

Burned Out? Stressed Out?

In the early studies during the 1940's, along with memory enhancement, some participants reported feeling a "mood enhancement" or increased ability to handle stress while taking pregnenolone. Some doctors believe pregnenolone may prove to be one of the most effective of all mood stabilizers. Current studies have shown that people with low levels of pregnenolone demonstrate symptoms of depression or are highly susceptible to showing symptoms of depression in the future. The National Institute of Mental Health claims clinically depressed people have subnormal levels of pregnenolone in their cerebral spinal fluid, and being a potent and essential neurosteroid, these lower levels could account for this mood disorder.

Our hormones play a key role in how our bodies and brains handle stressful situations. As we encounter stress—the children leave for college, a deadline at work, the in-laws in town—our hormones skyrocket to ward off the potentially injurious side effects of anxiety. One of the hormones found to be indispensable for mood stabilization and stress reduction is pregnenolone. Stress is toxic. This becomes obvious when you think of some of its manifestations: headaches, backaches, loss of memory and mental function, and despondency. The impact of stress on the body and mind can in itself deplete essential hormones and lead to premature aging and disease. In our fast-paced, information age, stress is inescapable, but with hormone supplementation, you can dodge its unhealthy effects as you grow older, or even—especially with pregnenolone—actually work better under its influence. In the 1940's and 50's, studies of factory workers under extreme pressure as a byproduct of being paid by the piece rather than by the hour showed, after supplementation of pregnenolone, that for many, stress levels dropped and productivity under such demands improved.

As pregnenolone produces adrenal steroids, it builds barricades of defense against stress. Remember in the DHEA chapter, its positive sway over the negative effects of stress. Pregnenolone, by producing DHEA, among other steroid hormones, can directly influence how we deal with stress. Supplementing your diet with pregnenolone can, therefore, reduce the harmful results of stress and, in some instances, reverse the effects the body and mind have already suffered from excessive exposure to tension and agitation.

Another feel-good benefit of pregnenolone is its ability to improve sleep quality and decrease the intermittent wakefulness that many older people experience. I can't tell you how many patients come to me with the complaint of fitful sleep. It's not abnormal to experience odd sleep patterns as you get older. Many people in their late forties find that their sleep habits have flip-flopped—they are sleepless at night and drowsy during the day. Aging has an antagonistic effect on our sleep, and it's important, when seeking the right path to a healthy future, to regain your youthful sleeping habits. Some doctors, myself included, believe that in our deepest recesses of sleep, our body revives itself from the stresses of the day. Deep stage IV sleep also releases human growth hormone, which when you read the HGH chapter you will understand exactly how beneficial this release is to our body and mind. Also this deep sleep releases cytokines which work to enhance our immune system. A good night's rest can do more than just help you function the next day, it actually helps you function healthily, for years to come.

As humans experience stress, cortisone levels skyrocket and become dangerous. At high levels, cortisone, whether natural or not, triggers unwanted and unhealthy effects. With each progressive year, stress increases, yet the protective levels of pregnenolone decline. One of the best ways to guard your physical and mental abilities against stress or depression is to replace your decreasing levels of pregnenolone. Stress can lead to depression, creating a domino effect and further diminishing hormone levels. There is no reason to be stressed or depressed about the effects of growing older when you have a potential antidote, a natural hormone replacement program, close at hand.

Above and Beyond

Pregnenolone's promise reaches far beyond the expectations of the scientists in the 1940's and as researchers continue to study this hormone, it may well hold out prospects for protecting against other complications associated with aging. Because pregnenolone promotes myelin formation for repair during nerve regeneration, scientists believe it may help victims of multiple sclerosis. It has also been used with spinal cord injury patients, and in some cases, when administered right after the injury, pregnenolone showed a possibility of inhibiting the chance of paralysis. These studies illustrate that pregnenolone may perhaps reduce the residual effects from an injury to the spinal cord.

Pregnenolone is a precursor to cortisone, which has been used extensively in treating arthritis. Pregnenolone has been found to be much safer and more cost effective than corticoids, salicylates, and gold—drugs sometimes used to treat arthritis pain—and it can be used at higher doses without producing toxic effects. Studies on the use of pregnenolone to treat joint pain, osteoarthritis, and gouty arthritis have been encouraging, with pain waning in less than a week.

Pregnenolone has also been known to reduce the signs of aging skin. Several studies have revealed that with a daily application of pregnenolone cream, wrinkles become less visible and skin is left radiant. Unfortunately, when the treatment is discontinued, the wrinkles return, but with prolonged and continued use, pregnenolone can help the skin stay hydrated, smooth, and refreshed.

As I mentioned earlier, studies since the 1940's have shown that pregnenolone is safe. The most likely side effects you will experience are amplified memory, added energy, a sense of well-being, greater mobility—the opposite of the typical side effects of aging.

I urge you to take into consideration pregnenolone as a must-have hormone in your tailored hormone program. It's a safe, natural alternative to many of the drugs meant to increase your memory or energy. It can help you retain the information you gather now and help you remember the information you gathered then. You can approach the next decades of your life, reassured that you've taken action against the age-related decline once foolishly believed a "natural" transition into your latter years.

Melatonin:
The Aging Loophole

After my hysterectomy I started waking up on and off at night and found that several nights a week I never fell completely asleep. I couldn't function during the day and felt on edge. My friend had a bottle of melatonin and gave me a week's supply. The first night I took it, I slept fantastic, and what's more incredible is that I never had to take prescription sleep-aids—I could find relief in something natural to my body's environment.
—Jaime, 54

What if I were to tell you that scientists and doctors may have discovered the aging loophole? What if I told you that a natural occurring sleep-aid is part of the longevity equation and should not be left out when considering hormone replacement therapy? Melatonin, which people have taken for years as a natural sleep aid, is the hormone that first opened physicians' eyes to the possibility of successfully treating aging as a disease. Although it has been under investigation since 1958, it has only been recently that its remarkable possibilities have been realized. Several books have been solely devoted to the subject of melatonin and what its supplementation means to the aging human body and mind. Perhaps the best known, comprehensive book on this hormone is The Melatonin Miracle by the well researched doctors William Regelson and Walter Pierpaoli. It's a must read for anyone curious about the ongoing discoveries being made regarding melatonin's functional importance in the human body. My goal in this particular chapter is to give you a good glimpse of the kind of lengths melatonin supplementation can go to concerning the topic of healthy aging. You'll understand from the studies I reference throughout this chapter that scientists have been able to demonstrate that melatonin can slow and reverse the aging processes in animals with genetic make-ups similar to that of humans. Because of the powerful evidence reaped from these studies, researchers are now looking into melatonin's potential as a powerful anti-oxidant, cancer inhibitor, immune system booster, and for its effects on ailments such as heart disease, AIDS, Alzheimer's, diabetes, and Parkinson's disease. No longer is melatonin known just for its sleep enhancing effects. Up-to-date science is also showing that the potential of this hormone may be vast in both its immediate and long-term capabilities.

Melatonin is derived from a chain of events starting with an amino acid called tryptophan, which is synthesized into serotonin, which then, by the action of two enzymes is catalyzed into melatonin. Once melatonin is released by the pineal gland, it goes into the local blood stream and then into the body's blood circulation where it has access to every bodily fluid and tissue. Its production is influenced primarily by the night-and-day cycle: in the light, production of melatonin decreases; with darkness, melatonin levels rise dramatically, causing us to become drowsy. Interestingly, unlike most hormones, melatonin does not necessarily need a receptor site; melatonin's small molecular structure and solubility allow it to permeate almost every cell in the body. Therefore, more than just a natural tranquilizer, melatonin seems to be the hormone-of-all-trades. Some researchers speculate that the exact amount of melatonin that reaches the DNA of every cell dictates which kinds of proteins to make. In fact, in 1994 in the *Journal of Biological Chemistry*, researchers found a specific receptor for melatonin directly in the nucleus of cells. This finding led to the conclusion, "A nuclear signaling pathway for melatonin may contribute to some of the diverse and profound effects of this hormone." Indeed, as the researcher concluded above, you too will more completely understand just how profound melatonin's actions are as you continue reading this chapter.

As you read this book and peruse the countless studies I cite about this new medical paradigm in aging prevention and probe deeper into how to preserve your own well-being as you grow older, you will find a large variant in how the replacement of hormones, and in this case, melatonin, are viewed. For as many researchers who have studies to back up the potential applications of melatonin, you will find others who are tentative about its use. Some believe we should wait to see what new tests may reveal, yet aging and its related ailments do not wait on hold while the final verdict about hormone replacement is being made. I don't know about you, but the studies throughout this chapter from some of the most prestigious medical journals have put my mind at ease, and I myself am not about to postpone my own quality of living while I wait for someone to make up their mind that through supplementation of melatonin, we can achieve a healthier aging. Above all, melatonin has proven itself, since 1958, to be effective with low toxicity. Studies have shown that it's safe and its benefits outweigh any possible side effects. I'm aware of why doctors are cautious about hormone replacement of any kind—it's considered "alternative medicine," but consider this while reading this book: What other alternative is out there? As I clinically uncover through reputable studies the reasons behind hormone replacement and its necessity to enjoying a healthier aging, you'll see that optimal replacement makes sense. In the case of melatonin, almost *50 years* of studies bolster its safety and clinical applications. I will argue with any critic that if fifty years isn't considered long term, I don't know what is.

Nature's Little Pacemaker

Melatonin is produced in the pineal gland—a tiny, pine-cone-shaped gland tucked deep within the human brain. Once thought of as an evolutionary leftover, the pineal gland became the center of research when it was discovered that it basically controls the hows and whens of aging. The pineal gland is believed to have evolved from primitive eye tissue and is known as the "third-eye." By stimulation of the day/night cycle, it adjusts the body rhythms accordingly, and helps keep the body acclimated to the environment, allowing it to adapt to such changes as traveling over several time zones in the space of a day. The pineal gland is also involved in the regulation of the endocrine system, the immune system, and the regulation of production of other hormones. Its job is one of maintaining a balance in the body, which it does through the synthesis and release of melatonin.

As we get older, the pineal gland atrophies, and the production and secretion of melatonin decreases. Some hypothesize that the body interprets this dip in melatonin production as a signal to age. As melatonin production wanes, other vital components of the body also begin to atrophy or waste away, such as the thymus gland, the spleen, and bone marrow. Both the thymus gland and spleen influence immune system function, while bone marrow impacts both the immune system and our bones' strength and health. As melatonin production drops, with it goes our regular sleep cycle, which influences immune health and hormonal secretion, like growth hormone, along with melatonin's stress and cancer-blocking capabilities—**it is then that** the body falls prey to various age-related ailments and inconveniences.

Doctors, therefore, myself included, believe that a crucial ingredient in the recipe for feeling young is maintaining an ongoing supply of the hormone a youthful pineal gland produces, which we can do by supplementing the body with melatonin. Many documented studies from laboratories around the world have confirmed the powerful link between the functions/secretions of the pineal gland and longevity.

Some of the most significant of these studies are illustrated by Dr. Walter Pierpaoli, one of the authors of <u>The Melatonin Miracle</u>. Dr Pierpaoli, an immunologist at the Biancalana-Masera Foundation for the Aged in Ancona, Italy, has spent years studying the effects of melatonin and the pineal gland on mammals. He first tested his hypotheses on several breeds of mice that naturally produce melatonin. The mice were in the range of nineteen months old, which converts to about sixty-five human years (the normal life span for these mice is about twenty-four months). Dr. Pierpaoli suspected that a group of mice given melatonin in their drinking water would remain healthier than a controlled group that received no melatonin supplementation at all. The doctor saw no change until the fifth month, when noticeable differences left the doctor and his staff amazed. His results seemed to exceed all expectations.

The mice given melatonin preserved their thick, shiny coats, clear eyesight, strong bones and muscle tone, and sexual activity. The others exhibited the normal but lamentable signs of aging: hair loss, lackluster fur, cataracts, poor digestion, and hampered mobility. The mice that had received no melatonin supplementation lived out their normal life span. The melatonin-supplemented mice lived six months beyond their expected life span (a twenty-five percent increase), and they lived in a more "youthful" state. In the words of Jo Robinson, co-author of <u>Melatonin: Your Body's Natural Wonder Drug</u>, with melatonin, the mice were able to die "young as late in life as possible."

Dr. Pierpaoli retested several times with the same results. He then decided to take his investigation several steps further and focus on melatonin's source—the pineal gland. If the pineal gland was really the "aging clock," it seemed possible that a young pineal gland would result in a young body as well. In 1990, with the expertise of Vladimir Lesnikov, a Russian researcher, Dr. Pierpaoli surgically swapped the pineal glands of mice aged four months (twenty human years) with mice aged eighteen months (sixty human years). They also performed a sham operation: they removed the pineal gland from another set of four-month and eighteen-month old mice, and replaced them again in the same mice, to determine that it was the exchanged pineal gland which caused the observed effects rather than the operation alone.

As the weeks wore on, the researchers were surprised to find that the mice seemed to level out. The old had indeed grown younger, rejuvenated by a pineal gland; meanwhile, the young mice with the old pineal glands aged at an increased rate. Within a few weeks, in fact, both groups of mice had reached the same "age" from opposite directions. Soon afterward, Dr. Pierpaoli and Mr. Lesnikov watched as the young mice with old pineal glands began to decline at a fast pace and actually died sooner than expected. The old mice with the young pineal glands eventually lived thirty percent longer than expected.

The mice that underwent sham operations lived normal lives with typical life expectancies of twenty-four months.

The above studies are truly remarkable and telling of the potential applications of melatonin in the human body. Since it's not likely that pineal gland swapping is a possibility in humans, melatonin supplementation is under review as a more plausible solution to the aging phenomenon. In the next segments, I would like to help you discover the vast applications of this basic yet often overlooked hormone. Like other hormones, melatonin can't stop time, but it can derail or delay many of time's debilitating effects. It may not be the most glamorous hormone, but I do believe it to be a necessary addition for everyone who is serious about their longevity program. As you read this next segment, you will understand how melatonin begins helping us toward a healthier aging by boosting our immune system.

On the Warpath

Keeping our immune system operating in top form is key to preventing illnesses and early death. The strength of our immune system directly impacts how our body fends off foreign invaders—from a simple flu bug to cancer cells. If we do nothing to help prevent it as we age, our immune system, like everything else, begins its own decline. As it does, it becomes much harder to ward off even common ailments like the flu or colds—someone sniffles near us, and we're off to bed for a week.

Via the secretion of melatonin, the pineal gland affects the thymus gland, the spleen, and bone marrow and each of these, in turn, affect the immune system's efficiency. In our younger days, our immune system had an uncanny way of eliminating harmful substances from our body. When approached by a foreign attacker, a young immune system creates an antibody that will remember it and be able to purge the body of it should it return again. As we get older, many elements of the immune system become unresponsive. Our antibody production and effectiveness diminishes, and an infection our bodies once recognized and fought off effectively is allowed to run rampant. How the absence of melatonin is related to the decline in our immune system is revealed by studies on animals that have shown time and time again that when the pineal gland is removed and melatonin synthesis is therefore inhibited, the subjects experience a kind of immunosuppression. Yet, when melatonin is restored orally, a healthy immune system is seemingly jump-started. Melatonin supplementation helps shore up our defenses on both fronts by improving our immune system's memory and strengthening its antibody response, allowing our immune system to function closer to the peak level we had at one time.

Not only do our antibodies fail us but our armed forces, the "killer" T-cells that fight off pathogens and foreign bodies, also wind down. This is aggravated by the atrophy of our thymus gland, which is involved in T-cell production and storage. Exploration into how melatonin works has demonstrated that physiological concentrations of melatonin can stimulate the release of opioid peptides (substances found naturally in the body that act on the brain to decrease sensation of pain) by activated T-helper lymphocytes. The researchers believed that the melatonin-induced immuno opioids lend themselves to the immunoenhancing and anti-stress effects seen in subjects supplemented with melatonin.

Another study showed that melatonin, when chronically injected into young mice or mice immunosuppressed by aging or under immunosuppressive treatment, was able to enhance the antibody response to a T-dependent antigen. The enhancement of antibody response was associated with increased induction of T helper cell activity and IL-2 production as evidenced in the groups of mice who needed the most help—the immunodepressed by aging or immunosuppressed mice. These observations suggest that melatonin may be successfully used in the therapy of immunodepressive conditions, like that seen in chemotherapy procedures and aging.

An interesting constituent Dr. Pierpaoli discovered in his experiments on pineal glands and mice was that the thymus gland, which was shrunken before, was restored to its original size when a new pineal gland was implanted. This lead to improved T-cell production and function, which meant increased power to fight off pathogens. There is also evidence (as seen in the study above) that melatonin can help restore thymus function and that melatonin enhances T-cell production. By enhancing T-cell production, melatonin can also help the body fight viruses—another vital factor in keeping the disease of aging in check. Melatonin's role in the immune system is supported by the evidence that there is a high relation of melatonin receptors in human T lymphocytes.

T-cells and the thymus gland also work to help eliminate the negative side effects of stress. When you're stressed, your susceptibility to infection heightens. The immune system breaks down under the pressure of chronic stress and the body opens up to a world of common colds and flues or, even worse, debilitating illnesses like heart disease or cancer. When exposed to high levels of stress the body produces corticosteroids, stress hormones that in high quantities can become harmful.

Melatonin can decrease the harmful effects of corticosteroids by reducing their levels back to normal, thus mitigating or preventing the excess damage these hormones can cause, as well as keeping T-cell production up. And as I mentioned before, melatonin has been seen to augment the substances in the human body that lessen pain and allow our bodies to cope and heal.

Stress is nothing to take lightly. Each passing decade adds new stresses to the old, while, paradoxically, as we age, many of our natural defenses deteriorate. Melatonin, which once naturally inhibited the effects of corticosteroids and enhanced the benefits of our endorphins (anti-pain and -anxiety chemicals), suddenly decreases and without melatonin to check them, corticosteroids levels may rise and wreak havoc on the body. Melatonin can help alleviate the effects and damage from stressors in our environment and be an important, natural tranquilizer.

Beyond melatonin's power as an immune system booster, melatonin is also being touted as a powerful antioxidant, and rightly so. Studies as current as 2001 show that melatonin's awesome free radical scavenging capabilities may help the mind as well as the body. Anti-oxidants are vital in combating what are known as "free radicals." Free radicals are unstable molecules that attack stable molecules in order to provide themselves with the electron they are missing. Although the life span of a free radical is short, its damage can be long lasting. Some doctors and scientists believe free radicals are the direct cause of aging, since they rip electrons from perfectly functioning atoms, causing degradation and disruption within a cell.

Antioxidants like vitamin E, vitamin C, glutathione, and melatonin block free radicals from robbing electrons from healthy atoms. Melatonin scavenges oxygen-centered free radicals and among the more powerful anti-oxidants, melatonin has been found to be the best hydroxyl scavenger. The hydroxyl radical is highly toxic and melatonin works by attaching to it to neutralize it by single electron transfer, resulting in a detoxified radical. It's important to note here that melatonin's actions as a free radical scavenger are not mediated by receptors, and this is why I call it the hormone-of-all-trades—it has actions above and beyond the duty of a hormone.

Examples of melatonin's potent antioxidant effects are seen in such studies like that of the 1993 report in which rats were given safrole, a carcinogen, either alone or paired with melatonin. Safrole causes nucleic acid damage in a DNA strand by producing oxygen radicals. The following results give melatonin high marks, when illustrating its possible use in controlling free radical damage:

> The amount of DNA damaged by safrole (300 mg/kg) was reduced by 41 percent even when the dose of safrole administered was 1,500 times greater than the dose of melatonin (0.2mg/kg). When the dose of melatonin (0.4 mg/kg) was doubled, DNA damage was reduced by 99 percent.

As you know, DNA is the map of our design and suffers the most from ionizing radiation due to oxidative stress. Melatonin shields the macromolecules, such as DNA, from injury, thus halting the process of disease that causes proliferate and degenerative changes. Because melatonin flows so easily in and out of cellular compartments, it is a constant and potent antioxidant. Melatonin, in fact, may guard against a number of conditions tied to oxidative stress like Alzheimer's disease, cancer, Parkinson's disease, multiple sclerosis, and rheumatoid arthritis. Proof of this can be seen in more current studies, which illustrate its effectiveness in fighting neuronal alterations due to oxidative processes. In 2001, a team of researchers illustrated that melatonin, above estrogen and vitamin E, had neuroprotective effects against kainic acid-induced damage in the hippocampus. The researchers concluded that, since kainic acid is believed to cause neuronal alterations due to oxidative processes, the free-radical scavenging properties of melatonin account for the protective effects seen within the study.

Melatonin has many receptor sites in the human brain and, as studies reveal over and over again, it may have a definitive purpose as a natural defense in many age-related degenerative diseases. Of course, its antioxidant applications are clear. Whether we can use this knowledge to fight off diseases like Parkinson's and Alzheimer's has yet to be seen. Fighting free-radical damage is a start in our quest for a healthier aging—and melatonin's worth in this arena is indisputable.

Where we stand with melatonin and other hormones on age-related diseases is still under investigation. Some hormones have proven themselves, without a doubt, to be, through supplementation, preventable methods in the aging process. Estrogen guards against heart disease and osteoporosis, and studies are also showing it has a protective effect against Alzheimer's in women; while testosterone, in both men and women, has shown to encourage heart and bone health, along with positive physical alterations like a positive muscle to fat ratio. As far as melatonin goes, I can only report what directions studies are pointing to, and the conclusions these studies seem to suggest to the aging dilemma. In the next segment you will see exactly what I mean. The next studies I cite only hint at what kinds of applications may be in store for melatonin in the future.

Cancer—A Common Foe of Aging

Because melatonin augments the immune response and battles against free radicals, it should be no surprise that it is also believed to be an inhibitor of tumor growth and useful as a supplement in cancer therapy. Some cancers are hormone dependent, yet melatonin may actually decrease this threat by regulating the output of estrogen and obstructing estrogen receptors on breast cells. As I have said, melatonin acts as a mediator to many other hormones. Because of this, melatonin can help protect against hormone dependent cancers. It has also been shown to indirectly attack breast cancer cells and impede prostate cancer cells.

There is also good news for cancer patients who endure harsh cancer treatments. A study performed by Dr. Paoli Lissoni at Geraldo Hospital in Milan, Italy, has shown that interleukin 2, coupled with melatonin, can actually be administered in a smaller dose, which greatly lessens the severe and painful side effects interleukin 2 has been known for. Other studies have illustrated that melatonin administered along with radiotherapy increased patients' life span than over those patients solely on radiotherapy.

Melatonin's cancer-obstructing benefits, along with its therapeutic benefits for cancer victims, are still under speculation. Since cancer still poses an illusive threat, alternative therapies are in the trial and error stage. We can only conclude from the large amount of data that melatonin has a place in this field of research and care. If you have cancer or cancer is in your family genes, before self-prescribing you will want to talk to your doctor about how melatonin may help you. I always suggest finding a doctor open to different methods of treatment, and if you have to pull out the studies, you will find them at the end of this book—they are there in black and white and they pose a good case when it comes to cancer and its different modes of therapies.

I've discussed melatonin's boundless effects on our immune system. It has a large amount of clinical data to support its use in the body as we get older and become susceptible to ailments of aging. Yet, although melatonin has far-reaching capabilities, nothing is as obvious as its utility as a sleep-aid.

Sleep: Nature's Tonic

Sometimes the best medicine is simply a good night's rest. Sleep has its own regenerating power that can do wonders at reconstructing the damage done during the waking hours. The only rest for the senses is deep sleep, and the only way to fall into that stage IV sleep is through the ebb and flow of melatonin. You will also learn at the end of the book that human growth hormone, our powerful healing hormone, is secreted during stage IV sleep. The lackluster sleep we experience as we get older influences our health in noticeable ways—bad concentration and irritable moods; and unnoticeable ways—our human growth hormone levels decline and we're more susceptible to pathogens.

The pineal gland is wired to a paired cluster of nerve cells above the optic chasm in the hypothalamus. At night, the darkness sends a message to this cluster of nerves, which then sends impulses to the pineal gland, which in turn, secretes melatonin. Melatonin causes the yawning, the droopy eyelids, the heavy limbs, and the yearning to curl up under the covers and sleep. Its levels rise tenfold at night, peaking at around two in the morning and stimulating stage IV sleep, the deepest sleep, where the body and mind recoup from daily stresses.

I personally take melatonin for this reason—out of the motivation to get a good night's sleep (I count all of its other side benefits as bonuses). What I have noticed as I get older, and as I'm sure you'll relate to, sleep is not as easy to come by as it was when I was in my youthful prime. I find myself tossing and turning without melatonin's aid, and the next morning and throughout the next day, I have a harder time concentrating. Melatonin's ability to promise a deep sleep, in itself, allows our bodies and minds to stay healthy. Laymen's proof of this is seen in our reaction to tossing and turning at night. Nights of sleeplessness can drastically inhibit our immune system, and to be perfectly honest with you, they can also inhibit our sense of humor and good will to others. Sleep is essential to staying healthy and happy, and melatonin is the elixir to a good night's rest.

With age comes a drop in melatonin production and with this drop also comes insomnia and sleep disorders often associated with age. Again, a lack of sleep can add to the stresses on the body and the immune system, contributing to the problems associated with age. Supplementing the diet with melatonin can be an effective treatment for insomnia in older patients. A 2000 study demonstrated that an age-related "melatonin deficiency state" creates the insomnia characterized in many older people and that this insomnia is treatable with the replacement of low doses of melatonin to the amplitude seen in young adults. The same researcher five years earlier also examined nine elderly insomniacs on melatonin supplementation. That study also demonstrated significant increases in sleep efficiency and decreases in nocturnal awakenings and sleep latency with the aid of melatonin supplementation.

Because melatonin controls the circadian rhythms, it can also reset the sleep cycle when it gets interrupted. Travelers have used melatonin for years to fight jet lag. By taking melatonin the first night you arrive in a new time zone, the circadian rhythms are forced to adjust at a faster rate. Those few days on vacation you've always set aside for "zombie-mode" can now be open to a world of opportunities.

Many people throughout the United States depend upon prescription sleep-aids to get through the night. These types of sleep-aids can have side effects, and what's worse, they can become addictive. Melatonin has neither of the above deterrents. It is safe, yet powerful, and non-addictive.

Is Melatonin for You?

Melatonin has proven to be one of the safest hormones you can take. Melatonin is metabolized quickly and the body only uses the amount it needs. Tests administering high doses to both mice and humans have indicated no toxic effects. In a human study, 6,000 mg (1000 mg over the recommended dose) was administered before bedtime for a month. Subjects reported an occasional headache or disorientation, but overall the study demonstrated that melatonin is generally harmless.

There are those who should not or do not need to supplement with melatonin. Most doctors and scientists agree that children have enough melatonin, and young adults, around the age of twenty, are experiencing their peak in melatonin output. Forty to forty-five may be the optimum age for beginning to use a melatonin supplementation. Only a doctor experienced in hormone replacement therapy can best fit your needs and answer your concerns regarding what kind and how much of hormone replacement is necessary.

Melatonin has gone through a battery of tests throughout the years without much show of toxicity or side effects. It has had quite the following, with some skeptics worried about the hype and mania over this over-the-counter drug. I believe the hype is qualified by peer-reviewed studies featured in some of the world's most prestigious medical journals. In January, 1997, the *New England Journal of Medicine* published the most extensive review of melatonin yet to appear in a conventional medical journal. This article extolled melatonin's powerful antioxidant effects, its potential for treating and preventing cancer, its immuno-enhancing properties, its potential to slow aging, and its power to induce better sleep and treat jet lag. Melatonin is a vital catalyst in both the endocrine and immune system functioning. It is a key to the thymus gland's maintenance and T-cell production, antibody efficiency, regulation of the circadian rhythm, and by its action as a powerful free radical scavenger. Most important, melatonin is one of the hormones shown time and again to turn back certain aspects of the "aging clock" in a way that prevents age-associated deterioration and may protect against age-related disease.

Estrogen:
The Genesis of Hormone Replacement

I had hot flashes that seemed to rip through me like a Saharan wind. I couldn't sleep and most times I felt like a zombie. Once my doctor prescribed me natural estrogen, the hot flashes disappeared after two days. It was a miracle.
—Janis, 48

Estrogen restored my sense of well-being. I remember after my hysterectomy how depressed I had become. I felt disconnected, like they took more than just my ovaries and uterus. It wasn't until I took natural hormones that I realized I was missing something. I felt alive again.
—Macey, 53

In a very real sense, it was menopause that opened the door to total hormone replacement therapy.

For more than forty years, doctors have prescribed estrogen to women suffering from menopausal symptoms such as hot flashes, vaginal dryness, problems with concentration and anxiety, and insomnia. Estrogen replacement therapy proved to be so effective that some women continued taking the hormone even after menopause had passed. These women felt better, looked better, and—once doctors and scientists began to look into it—these women were *doing* better. Aside from any cosmetic benefits—stronger hair, smoother skin, and improved muscle tone—estrogen also decreased their risk of osteoporosis, heart disease, and colon cancer. It was unanticipated benefits like these that led to doctors taking a closer look at the role hormones play in health and aging.

Women, along with their doctors, are now realizing that menopause is not a period in life to be endured and ignored as a natural transition into old age or the beginning of the end. Instead, it is a condition that can easily be transformed as a rite of passage into a woman's second adulthood. Women are now living 30 to 40 years beyond menopause, therefore this time in their life, menopause and postmenopause, needs critical attention and research. For women to avoid a dramatic slide during and after menopause, they must find the resources that make that avoidance possible. Estrogen and progesterone are the resources and are not only effective but have been shown to exceed women's expectations of feeling as effectual and energetic as they did prior to menopause.

Estrogen is an essential hormone that not only confronts the uncomfortable symptoms of menopause but also helps maintain a healthy and youthful environment within the body. Hormone replacement therapy is a very safe and effective treatment against the numerous possible complications age carries with it. Natural estrogen replacement, as opposed to synthetic or altered estrogens, carries with it a genuine ally in bolstering bone health, improving heart vasodilation, and defending the mind against the process that makes Alzheimer's disease possible. It's a woman's best safeguard against the diseases that accompany age. In this chapter, I would like to increase your awareness about the insurmountable proof of natural estrogen's benefits to the female body. The benefits *do* outweigh any risk you may have encountered. I would like to start with the benefits and then discuss the risks and the major differences between the natural and synthetic forms of estrogen and progesterone. It's important for a woman to be educated as she enters her second adulthood. Since women are living longer lives, I want those lives to be absent of bone loss, heart complications, and Alzheimer's disease. I believe in and stand by the powerful benefits that natural estrogen provides for the female body. When you're through reading this chapter, I hope you too will understand how natural hormones support the body in and after middle age. I also hope to clear up any confusion between synthetic and natural estrogens. It's not just a matter of semantics but also a matter of one's optimal health. My goal is that you, as a curious woman on the cusp or perhaps suffering from menopause or its after effects, can use this book as resource in your pursuit for a more healthy and enjoyable way of living.

Not Just a Matter of Semantics

There seems to be much confusion over the wording in hormone replacement therapy. I'm sure you've heard the adjectives "natural" or "synthetic," but these words become interchangeable and it becomes a matter of source rather than true definition. I understand this mix-up, and as a doctor of longevity medicine I hope to clear up any misinterpretation that you may have read or been told by your doctor. When I use the phrases "natural estrogen replacement" or "natural progesterone replacement," or simply combine the two into the phrase "natural hormone replacement," I'm talking about bio-identical hormones, or hormones that match the chemical make-up of the hormones your body produces naturally. Unfortunately, the term "natural" has been used loosely, and some patients as well as doctors believe "natural" refers to products derived from plants (yams) or animals (horses). Just because they come from a natural source, doesn't mean they're good for the body.

Many fruits, vegetables, grains, nuts, herbs, and spices, called phytoestrogens, have minor estrogenic capabilities. Some companies purport that these "natural" products can eliminate menopausal symptoms. The truth is that even the strongest phytoestrogens have about one to two percent the estrogen potency of human estrogens. Yams seem to be the most popular and recommended source of "natural" estrogen supplementation. In health food stores and advertised all over the Internet are wild yam creams that can supposedly cure menopausal symptoms and menstruation difficulties. Although the Mexican wild yam can be synthesized by a biochemist into a variety of hormones: DHEA, progesterone, testosterone, and the three estrogens, the human body does not have the capabilities, or cofactors, to convert this precursor into the essential hormones stated above. If you consume wild yams or rub wild yam cream on your arm you've really done nothing to alleviate your menopausal symptoms.

Conjugated hormones derived from pregnant mares' urine, under the brand name Premarin, are widely used by women and clinics across the United States. Simply put, these are equine hormones, and they cannot fully match or work within the human female body. It's considered natural because it is not synthesized in a laboratory. I personally believe that there is nothing natural about supplementing a female human with female horse hormones. Later, in the Synthetic verses Natural segment, I will discuss exactly why Premarin is not the ideal choice for the female body.

Bio identical hormones are indistinguishable from human hormones. Their source may not *sound* as natural, since they are synthesized in a laboratory from soy to match the chemical make-up of naturally occurring human hormones. But, I ask you, what is more natural than something that is formulated to fit your body? As I talk about estrogen replacement throughout this chapter, and its benefits, I'm referring to bio-identical hormones. I firmly believe that it's a disservice to give patients, who are seeking methods to sequester the youth and vitality they once possessed, chemically altered estrogen replacement, or estrogen that does not naturally fit the female body.

Estrogen: The Whats, Hows, and Whys

Although men convert a small amount of testosterone into estrogen to meet certain bodily needs, estrogen is primarily a female hormone produced in the ovaries and adrenal glands. The female body produces three types of estrogen: estrone, estradiol, and estriol. Estradiol is the strongest of all the estrogens and the most abundant during the reproductive years. After menopause, estrone takes center stage as the predominant estrogen. Estriol is the metabolic byproduct of the two with the weakest estrogenic effect. These three estrogens, through direction of the hypothalamus, work in unison throughout a woman's life to protect her in her adolescent years, her reproductive years, and after menopause throughout her latter years by way of supplementation. Estrogen supplementation increases a woman's likelihood for a long life by balancing HDL and LDL levels, maintaining calcium in the bone tissue, preserving the blood vessel's youthful elasticity, and by keeping the arteries free and clean of the deadly plaque that causes heart disease.

Unfortunately, as with the hormones previously discussed, levels of all three estrogens plummet drastically with the onset of menopause. As the ovaries begin to shut down, estradiol levels that once peaked at 200 picograms per milliliter can plunge to levels barely reaching 30 picograms per milliliter. The menopausal process does not happen overnight, nor does it take place in a year. The hormonal changes actually take place over a duration sometimes referred to as the "climacteric," a two-to-fifteen-year period that spans from perimenopause to postmenopause. During this time frame, a female's hormones become erratic, causing abnormal physical and emotional symptoms. Perimenopause onset is signaled by irregular periods and sporadic hot flashes. These symptoms are directly spurred by the slackening of estrogen levels. Menopause takes place when the cessation of the monthly cycle occurs longer than a twelve-month period. The symptoms that started during the primary part of menopause usually carry over into the latter part of menopause, and estrogen drops twenty percent of where it once resided during a woman's reproductive years.

Menopause is not the only hormone-buster that women need to worry about. Many women undergo hysterectomies, meaning that the cessation of their periods is brought on surgically rather than naturally. These women undergo a partial or full hysterectomy, meaning either the uterus is removed while the ovaries are spared, or there is a removal of both. When both are removed the women are thrown into a sudden, surgical menopause and some, not all, women suffer from menopausal symptoms immediately. Whether or not these women negatively experience the sudden cessation of their hormones, they should supplement their bodies with estrogen, progesterone and testosterone, perhaps even more so than women who experience a more gradual hormonal drop. If you're a woman who has undergone a hysterectomy, you may have noticed a dramatic change—especially coupled with the trauma of a radical surgery. The quote by "Macey" at the beginning of this chapter is how many women feel after a full hysterectomy, and too many of these women are placed on antidepressants rather than the natural hormones that will most likely quell the side effects. Yet it's not just side effects that you should worry about. Without these vital and health sustaining hormones, women who have experienced full hysterectomies are in just as much danger as women who have gone through a naturally occurring menopause, in that they too are susceptible to heart disease, osteoporosis, or age related dementia. Not to mention their quality of life may also experience a severe dip. Women who retain their ovaries and only undergo a partial hysterectomy continue to have hormone production until the traditional menopause takes place, although they too may need hormone replacement.

With or without ovaries, it's crucial for women to balance their hormones and keep them at optimal levels. Regardless of how or when you experience menopause, the years after depend on the supplemental benefits of natural estrogen and progesterone. As you read on you'll more fully understand why.

The Menopause Cure-all

In 1989 I was going crazy. I was forty-five and my head was coming apart. I screamed at my kids and my lover and wept at nothing. I was a walking catalogue of symptoms. I have always been a little neurotic but it never bothered me before. Now I felt out of register. I was lost inside an alien body, monstrous, too large, off-balance. I got dizzy. My hands tingled a lot. Rushes of nameless horror came over me. One day while watching a football game I realized that I was about to die, that it was meaningless even to try to draw breath, and after a moment found myself sitting there, holding my breath like a woman underwater.

—Cecilia Holland
<u>Hot Flashes: Women Writers on the Change of Life.</u>

When estrogen levels decrease, usually during a woman's mid to late forties, menopause sets in and some women face a whole spectrum of uncomfortable and unsettling physical and emotional symptoms. These often include vasomotor changes (hot flashes), vaginal dryness, insomnia, difficulty concentrating, weight gain, and alterations in skin and hair texture. These changes, of course, precipitate and aggravate the emotional element of menopause: as a woman sees and feels her body becoming unfamiliar and older, feelings of insecurity, depression, and anxiety may set in. These feelings are mostly temporary since after menopause, most of the troublesome physical symptoms disappear. Their disappearance, however, is anticlimactic in the wake of the increased risks of cardiovascular disease, stroke, osteoporosis, and Alzheimer's. I believe it is no coincidence, therefore, that estrogen is the most prescribed medication in America, with more than 10 million women benefiting from estrogen replacement therapy today.

Seventy-five percent of all perimenopausal, menopausal, and postmenopausal women suffer from hot flashes—a sudden shock of warmth followed by perspiration and sometimes heart palpitations. For some women, these sudden jolts of heat are minor and few and far between, but for others they can be absolutely debilitating, interrupting their normal day-to-day activities or disrupting their sleep at night. We're not exactly sure of the mechanism behind this surge of heat, but we are positive it is directly linked to the sudden shortage of estrogen. Women report that it strikes without warning but is gone before they can crack a window or grab a piece of paper to fan off with. Although it is quick, it can be disorienting or embarrassing in front of coworkers or friends. This is the main reason estrogen replacement therapy got underway in the first place, so women could ride out menopause without feeling its bothersome symptoms. Estrogen supplementation eliminates these flare-ups in a matter of days, restoring a woman's self-confidence and composure in everyday situations. Unfortunately, too many women used estrogen as a temporary cure for menopause, rather than a long-term means to increase the quality of life beyond menopause. What these women miss out on far outreaches the convenient quick-fix estrogen offers during menopause.

Along with hot flashes and night sweats (which cause insomnia), some women also experience alarming irregularities in their period. For most women their period is the telltale sign that they are healthy, but during perimenopause the monthly cycle goes awry. Periods can range sixty to twenty-five days apart, some periods are light, while others are heavy and prolonged. Do not be alarmed, your body is adjusting to its sudden lack of hormones.

Many women patients also complain of mood swings, and this symptom seems to receive more press than any other trait of the menopausal process. I remember, in particular, a woman sitting in my office with a balled up Kleenex in one hand and a bottle of prescription mood-stabilizers in the other. I'll call her "Rebecca." She had been put on Prozac to curtail her "mood disorder" when she was forty-five. At the age of forty-six she was sitting in my office at the urging of a co-worker with tears streaming down her face. Rebecca believed she was doomed, and her husband believed he had married Dr. Jeckyl and Mr. Hyde. After having her blood drawn and tested, I was able to assure Rebecca she did not have a split personality, she was simply lacking the proper levels of the hormone essential for her emotional health. After three weeks on a combination of estriol and estradiol, she visited me without her Kleenex and the hopelessness that seemed to enshroud her less than a month before. She mentioned that she felt as if a heavy wool blanket had been removed from her shoulders, like she could breath again.

Since estrogen interacts with beta-endorphins in the brain, (the neuropeptides that curtail pain while enhancing a sense of well-being) the amount of its levels in the body influence how a woman will view and react to her surroundings. Good moods and balanced emotions in the beginning of the menstrual cycle are attributed to estrogen's high levels. As a woman gets older and estrogen levels begin to decline, it's no surprise her mood goes down the tubes with it. With the erratic aspect of a woman's hormones during perimenopause, and the intersection of these crazed hormones with the ongoing process of life, it is no wonder that some women are overwhelmed by depression. For some women this is an already hectic era in their lives. Children are leaving the home, marriages, therefore, adjust, and parents are getting older and more feeble. The added emotional irritation in conjunction with the physical loss of youth can cause mild to moderate depression. Estrogen has proven itself to be a veritable adversary to the menopausal blues. In a double-blind, placebo-controlled study, women, supplemented with estrogen and progesterone, demonstrated an increase of well-being via their results on the Profile of Adaptation to Life test and a decrease in depression measured via their results on the Beck Depression Inventory.

Other symptoms, vaginal dryness and infection, can also be side stepped with estrogen supplementation. Since the entire genitourinary tract is lined with estrogen receptors, an estrogen deficiency creates negative changes in the vagina's environment. The mucosa do not, as readily, lubricate the vagina when sexually aroused, compromising the prospect of intimacy. It is just too painful and therefore, uninviting. I've had many patients tell me they felt guilty because they no longer desired sex, and along with the mood swings they felt they were on totally different planets than their husbands. A patient of mine told me she felt "alienated" not just from her husband, but from the most common daily activities like taking a shower, tying her shoe, making toast.

Not only does the mucosa stop functioning correctly, but a woman loses epithelial cells, causing the walls of the uterus to become thinner and thinner. This is called "vaginal atrophy," where the walls become insubstantial and the actual vagina becomes shorter and narrower. A woman at thirty may have fifty to sixty vaginal layers, while a woman of eighty years of age may only have eight. As the skin thins, the cells that maintained the delicate acidic balance become more alkaline, putting the vagina at risk for bacteria to cause infection. The thinning also leaves the vagina disposed to chafing, leaving a woman prone to developing urinary and vaginal infections. Estrogen limits this effect by restoring vaginal tone and elasticity. It increases blood flow and enhances the vagina's lubricating ability. Sex is a natural human hunger, and menopause should *not* be the final curtain on such an essential and enjoyable aspect of a woman's life.

Another awesome capability of estrogen therapy is the positive influence it has on the skin. We have heard the phrases, "aging gracefully" or she "ages well." The cardinal physical signs of aging reside in the skin, which becomes dry and thin, and therefore wrinkles. This especially happens to women after menopause. How estrogen therapy helps women maintain thicker, healthier skin is quite simple. Estrogen stimulates the production of hyaluronic acid which helps hold water and moisture in the inner layer of skin, supporting the outer layer. This support allows the skin more elasticity while maintaining its firmness. Researchers in a 2000 study found that women supplemented with estradiol had better skin texture than women on a placebo. Tissue changes were evaluated by skin biopsy of the left upper arm at baseline and then again after six months of treatment. They found an exciting increase of collagen content. This is truly rousing news to the disheartened woman who's noticing her skin beginning to sag and the wrinkles beginning to accumulate. You no longer have to spend your life's savings on creams and sprays, estrogen naturally tightens and adds firmness to sagging skin.

Natural estrogen inhibits the common symptoms a large number of women feel when passing through the menopausal years. Forty years of successful therapy has proven, beyond a shadow of a doubt, that for many women, hot flashes, insomnia, mood swings, and vaginal dryness can be eliminated through estrogen supplementation. What estrogen does for the body before and during menopause is truly amazing, but what should be my primary concern as a doctor, and your uppermost interest as a maturing woman, are the years after menopause, when aging without estrogen can truly undermine your health. By breaking aging's chain of events through estrogen supplementation, you can avoid such illnesses as osteoporosis, heart disease, and Alzheimer's disease.

Osteoporosis: A Breakthrough for Healthy Bones

Uncomfortable side effects are only the beginning when it comes to troubles that can follow menopause. This is one reason I recommend that women include estrogen in their personal hormone regimen even after menopausal symptoms have disappeared.

For example, the rapid loss of bone mass after menopause has been directly linked with declining levels of estrogen. Science has now uncovered estradiol's important role in bone formation and has discerned receptor sites for estrogen in the female's skeletal structure. Estrogen is also important to the body's ability to utilize calcium, an essential ingredient for healthy bones. In these ways as well as others, estrogen has demonstrated a clear-cut benefit for preventing and treating osteoporosis.

Bone is dynamic tissue and each year 10 percent of it turns over, meaning new bone replaces the old. Women hit their peak bone mass about the age of thirty-five. From there on, although the bones still rebuild, women lose more bone than they're able to construct. As women age, their bodies process less new bone for old bone. The inner part of the bone, the trabecular bone, gets thinner while the outer bone, the cortical bone, retains its original shape. A hollowing occurs, and bones become brittle. In human bodies, cells called osteoclasts and osteoblasts continually tear down and rebuild bones. (Osteoclasts tear down old bone while osteoblasts build new.) As we age, the osteoclasts start outworking the bone-building osteoblasts, and we begin losing bone mass. For women, however, this loss can double, or even quadruple, from about 1 percent per year to 2-4 percent during the decade following menopause. The result is osteoporosis, "porous bones." Osteoporosis is more or less a silent disease that is usually undetected until after the damage has been done. About 24 million Americans suffer from osteoporosis, and 80 percent of those are women, especially older women. While osteoporosis itself does not kill, it cripples a woman's ability to live a healthy and active lifestyle. In some cases, complications arise after injuries such as hip fractures, which do kill a substantial number of osteoporosis sufferers in the United States each year.

There are certain bones that seem more easily lured into osteoporatic loss. The hip and wrist become fragile and easily fracture under the influence of osteoporosis. Also, osteoporosis causes the vertebral bone, the bone in your back, to collapse in on itself, resulting in a hunching over, or what is referred to as "dowager's hump." What is scary about this is that it usually takes four to five crushed vertebrae for a person to become aware of this debilitating and advanced disease.

The good news is that natural estrogen can cut a woman's risk of osteoporosis in half by decreasing the rate of bone loss. Estrogen fine tunes the process of bone remodeling by stimulating the release of calcitonin and vitamin D. Calcitonin, from the thyroid gland, inhibits osteoclasts, which slows down remodeling, maintaining adequate bone mass. Vitamin D helps the body absorb calcium from food and stimulates the kidneys to reabsorb calcium from the urine. This is one of the unexpected benefits doctors discovered for women who were taking estrogen for menopausal symptoms. In what is called the *PEPI Trials* (Postmenopausal Estrogen/Progestin Interventions), with results published recently in the *Journal of the American Medical*

Association, researchers tested five different treatments: a placebo; estrogen by itself; or estrogen with one of three progesterone regimens. After a three-year trial period, they assessed the results by measuring the bone mineral density at the hip and spine. "People who were taking the placebo lost about 3 percent of their bone density over the three years of study," Robert Marcas, Medicine Professor and director of study at Stanford University stated. "Women who took estrogen had a gain, on average, of 5 percent of bone density at their spine and about 2.5 percent at their hip over three years. Furthermore, 97 percent of the women who were treated had no bone loss at the spine, and 95 percent of women treated had no bone loss at the hip."

Another test conducted in 1985 called *The Study of Osteoporotic Fractures* (SOF) followed 9,704 women over sixty-five for seven years. The researchers found that the women using estrogen had 60 percent fewer wrist fractures, 40 percent fewer hip fractures, and 35 percent fewer nonspinal fractures as compared with women who did not supplement their diet with estrogen.

Osteoporosis can be a disabling disease. Women diagnosed with it find themselves concerned about their safety during certain activities they once considered normal. Once bones become too brittle, stepping off a curb or twisting in the most common way can cause a hip fracture. Osteoporosis is what I call "the second-guessing disease." But here is something you don't have to second-guess over—estrogen is a boon for the bone. Not only does it have its own receptor sites within the bone, estrogen oversees and puts into action the body's skeletal blueprint, a never ending construction project. Estrogen allows a woman to climb stairs, open a jar of pickles, or pick up her grandbaby without a second thought or feelings of trepidation.

Since women are at a higher risk for osteoporosis than men, especially thin, smaller boned Caucasian and Asian women, they need to take the proper precautions and include estrogen in their health maintenance regimen. It is first-line therapy that should be started in the perimenopause stage and continued throughout a woman's lifetime. Estrogen not only defines the curves on a younger woman's body, it also defines a matured woman by allowing her to stand taller and stronger as she ages and begins the adventure into the second half of her life.

Harnessing Heart Disease

Another pleasant surprise that doctors discovered is that women taking estrogen can cut their risk of heart disease by as much as *50 percent*. Estrogen's heart healthy attributes were discovered over forty years ago when doctors observed that women who had their ovaries removed became as susceptible to heart disease as men. Heart disease is a minor threat to younger women, but once they pass through menopause—and estrogen levels dip—heart disease becomes the number one killer of both men *and* women. Heart disease is no longer a male dominated disease and currently, almost *half* of all women die of heart disease in America. It's a middle-aged woman's most formidable enemy.

There are many facets that contribute to whether or not a woman will suffer from heart disease, although it seems more than just a coincidence that a woman's risk for heart disease escalates year after year as her estrogen levels continue to wane. Of course, other elements factor into whether or not a woman will suffer from heart complications. There are reasons behind why doctors have you fill out that long questionnaire before they treat you. Heredity plays a huge role in how your body will react to age and how a doctor should approach your specific type of aging. Aging is a personal matter. By assessing your past and that of your parents, a doctor will have some semblance of whether or not you will suffer from the atherosclerotic process or whether or not high LDL levels will be something of concern—both of which can be assuaged with the proper supplementation of natural estrogen.

Adult-onset diabetes increases a person's risk of cardiovascular disease. Diabetes actually doubles a woman's chance of developing heart disease. Estrogen increases insulin sensitivity, stopping short of adult onset diabetes. When insulin resistance occurs, the body makes up for it by creating more insulin. This overproduction can cause increased plaque formation in the blood vessels while increasing the chemical endothelin-1 that causes blood vessels to constrict. Mounting evidence shows that the presence of estrogen decreases the incidence of diabetes and thus decreases damage to and constriction of the blood vessels. *The Nurses' Health Study* reported, among other health advantages, that women who took estrogen had a twenty percent decrease in the incidence of diabetes.

Above and beyond estrogen therapy, women should look to a good diet and exercise regimen, combined with quitting smoking to lower their risks of heart disease. Smoking and weight are large contributors to heart disease and, I might add, something within a person's control. You make the choice whether to smoke or eat unwisely and not exercise. Smoking actually triples the risk of heart disease because it increases the oxidation of LDL and promotes vessel spasms. These spasms alter blood transportation to the heart, and eventually starve it of its life source. Obesity (being 20 percent over target weight) causes forty percent of heart complications in women.

Estrogen works in a number of ways to help reduce the risk of heart disease. For one, estrogen can help lower LDL (low density lipoprotein), "bad cholesterol," while raising HDL (high density lipoprotein), the "good cholesterol." Estrogen may also help protect the heart and arteries through its effect as a free radical scavenger. Some doctors and scientists believe that if we were able to effectively master free radical damage, we could add years to a human's life. Like vitamins E and C, estrogen acts as a powerful antioxidant and limits the oxidative damage to the arteries that causes plaque.

A 1995 study followed the heart progress of 7,610 women housed at Leisure World, a retirement village. The study observed women, mean age around seventy-three, who were either on estrogen or who had never used the hormone. The women on estrogen were protected from fatal and nonfatal heart attacks, while the women without were at *severe* risk. The women on estrogen had half the amount of fatalities due to heart failure as the women who had never benefited from its therapy.

Another study illustrated that levels of homocysteine, the amino acid considered a risk factor for vascular occlusion, were much lower in women who naturally had higher levels of estrogen or women who participated in an estrogen replacement program. Dr. Martha Savaria Morris and colleagues looked at the homocysteine levels of women of all different ages. What they found was that younger women or pregnant women who had higher estrogen levels, had lower homocysteine levels. They found this to also be the case in postmenopausal women who took estrogen supplements. Older women who did not take estrogen had homocysteine levels comparable to that of men their own age. These results validated the theory that estrogen somehow helped alter the levels of the amino acid linked to heart disease and therefore lowered the actual opportunity a woman had for heart problems.

Estrogen seems the mainstay, or backbone, to heart health. Many women who avoid hormone replacement for its purported risks are on a headlong journey toward heart complications. Natural estrogen replacement therapy makes a powerful argument for itself when it has proven time and again that it takes many recourses to stave off heart disease. It has been found that high doses of estrogen injected directly into a woman's arteries will dilate them, providing the proper amount of oxygenation to tissues. Beyond this, it has been shown without a doubt that women taking estrogen add years to their lives. A 2001 issue of the *American Journal of Epidemiology* reported the findings of the twelve-year *Cancer Prevention Study II*. Here, 300,000 postmenopausal women, who were cancer and cardiovascular disease free when they first enrolled, were followed and assessed. The women taking estrogen had a pronounced lower mortality rate than the women who never used estrogen. The comparison was most notable in regards to cardiovascular mortality, which was reduced by 30 percent in women who benefited from estrogen therapy. The gap was more noticeable in women who had lower body mass indexes and who were also taking estrogen. Their mortality rate dropped by fifty percent. This just goes to show that estrogen replacement coupled with a good diet and exercise regimen gives you that extra edge on longevity.

Other studies have shown that estrogen not only staves off heart disease but can also be used as a treatment of women who are already suffering from its debilitating blow. Women with established coronary artery disease benefit from estrogen supplementation and certain studies have shown that estrogen replacement therapy can reduce the risk of death or further cardio events by a brilliant 50 to 90 percent.

All of these life saving aspects of estrogen are only derived as long as a woman supplements her diet with the hormone. Only months after a woman ends her estrogen replacement compliance, do the risks again escalate. With the statistics of heart disease mortality as they are and the proof-positive results of estrogen therapy, I think it's startling that so many women lack vital knowledge about this life-saving hormone. Too many women are not reaping the benefits of this natural therapy. Your heart has been shielded by estrogen for the years before menopause, and as I showed in the studies above, without estrogen to fine-tune the complex workings of the heart, the vessels harden (atherosclerosis), plaque forms, and diabetes and stroke gain a firmer ground. Estrogen is perhaps the most vital part in maintaining a woman's healthy heart. In matters of the heart, estrogen replacement therapy has illustrated an impressive track record—so impressive that both the American Heart Association and the American College of Cardiology have issued guidelines recommending that physicians take into account using estrogen replacement therapy as a means to prevent or treat cardiovascular disease.

Brain Food

As research continues into the role hormones play in our bodies and the potential benefits of hormone replacement, scientists are confirming again and again that when it comes to hormones, what's good for the body is good for the brain. Although estrogen was never meant to be a preventative method or treatment for dementia, what studies have found are nothing short of exciting. Women on estrogen therapy often report an improvement in mood and feeling of well-being. They also sense an increase in their memory. Science is showing that this stems from more than just the relief that comes with treating the symptoms of menopause.

It's interesting that some women who have never had a problem with depression feel a sudden shift in the opposite direction with the onset of menopause. This is not surprising since estrogen is the body's own natural mood stabilizer. The pharmaceutical industry has formulated antidepressants, like Prozac and Zoloft, which do what optimal levels of estrogen have done all along—inhibit the serotonin-absorbing enzyme, monoamine oxidase (MAO), and allow the neurotransmitter serotonin to travel freely and elevate the mood. Estrogen, indeed, works on mood health in three different ways: it frees up tryptophan, a natural amino acid that transforms into serotonin in the brain; it decreases MAO activity; and it helps serotonin travel throughout the bloodstream by helping it "stick" to the surface of platelets. Many of my patients have attested to a returned optimistic outlook while on estrogen therapy and numerous studies have validated their claims. A patient of mine, "Esther," had been on Premarin for five years, after her hysterectomy. She couldn't put her finger on exactly why she felt so bad but she knew she felt despondent and irritable. She thought maybe she should be on an anti-depressant, and the magazines she read and commercials she watched at night seemed to validate her self-diagnosis. What "Esther" didn't realize until she visited me is that her body was not meshing with her prescribed horse estrogen. When I placed her on natural estrogen and progesterone, she noticed a dramatic change. She actually cared about what was going on inside and around her. She suddenly felt a part of her environment rather than alien to it. This is the reason behind hormone replacement therapy and the reason why doctors should treat patients, to make them feel healthier and happier.

In 1994, a European study used five hundred postmenopausal women to qualify what life after menopause was like. The women were on either of two drugs: Veralipride, a popular European drug used to subdue hot flashes, or estrogen. The women then answered a battery of five different questionnaires: The Global Women's Health Questionnaire, The Psychological General Well-Being Index, a sleep-problem questionnaire, a sexual-behavior questionnaire, and a questionnaire that evaluated their social life. Ninety-one percent of the women on estrogen answered "good" to "very good" to the questions in direct correlation with their quality of life, while only fifty percent of the women solely on Veralipride indicated they felt any increase in well-being or emotional health.

Estrogen and the brain have been cohorts since the very beginning. In the womb, maternal estrogen formulated and protected the fetus' brain. Later, estrogen stimulated memory and recall through certain neural receptors. Studies have shown that estrogen is involved in the synthesis of acetylcholine, one of the brain's most important chemical neurotransmitters; the production of brain cells; and the general, overall neural development and health. The brain is a developing organ that has the ability to grow or recede. As we grow older and our life sustaining hormone levels decrease, the tendency of the brain to recede is more common. What I mean by "recede" is that on the surface of the cells in the brain are fine structures called dendrites that branch out into dendritic spines which communicate with other cells. As the years creep on, the number of dendrites and dendritic spines decrease, and memory suffers in consequence. Estrogen actually protects this deterioration of the brain from happening. Not only this, but estrogen can increase the growth of dendrites and their spines, increasing communication between the cells and enforcing memory and learning retention. Countless studies have demonstrated estrogen's positive effects on memory and learning, as well as other mental processes.

Since women make up 72 percent of the population over the age of eighty-five, and nearly half of this group suffers from Alzheimer's disease, researchers are now taking a hard look at how estrogen may also reduce the risk of Alzheimer's disease. A study out of the University of Southern California showed that among 2000 subjects, the incidence of Alzheimer's was 40% lower among longtime estrogen users than women who had never taken estrogen. Other studies indicate that estrogen therapy may help delay the onset of Alzheimer's or lessen the severity of its effects.

I already mentioned that estrogen increases the enzyme necessary for the synthesis of acetylcholine, a chemical neurotransmitter that is involved in memory and the enzyme that happens to be abnormally low in Alzheimer's patients. Estrogen interacts with acetylcholine to protect the neurons from the ravages of age and helps foster new connections among nerve cells in the hippocampus, building bridges of communication that Alzheimer's disease would normally tear down.

There are a few distinctive features of Alzheimer's disease. Although it is normal for neurons to gradually decrease with age, in an Alzheimer's victim the rate of loss is significantly greater, especially in regions of the brain associated with memory and learning. Also doctors have found "neurofibrillary tangles" and B-amyloid, a build up of proteins, referred to as "neuritic (senile) plaque." The plaque damages the tissues by stimulating the neurofibrillary tangles or perhaps by programming cell death—no one quite knows exactly the progression or cause of Alzheimer's disease.

Mounting evidence has shown that women are three times more likely to develop the dreaded "forgetting" disease, and this likelihood rears its ugly head only after menopause robs the body of estrogen. Barbara Sherwin, a psychologist of Montreal's McGill University, studied the effect of estrogen supplementation on women who had previously had their ovaries removed and therefore suffered from estrogen deficiency. The women who took estrogen supplements could more easily learn and recall pairs of words compared to the women on a placebo. Interestingly, the positive effect on memory only affected verbal recollection rather than visual recollection. Although these tests may seem limited as far as real world application goes, it is important to understand how estrogen elevates memory in regard to Alzheimer's disease.

Another larger scale study performed at the University of Southern California also showed estrogen's positive feedback in regard to Alzheimer's disease. Researchers examined the medical histories of 2,418 women who had resided in a retirement home over the span of eleven years, 1981-1992. In reviewing the menstrual records of the deceased women, the researches noticed that the women who had taken supplements of estrogen were forty percent less likely to have developed the disease. The longer they had taken the hormone, the better chance the women had of never experiencing the blanking out of memories.

Certain studies have shown that with estrogen, even temporary estrogen supplementation, Alzheimer's can be put off for years, and in the scheme of things, every additional year counts. Interestingly, even women who took estrogen for four months to control symptoms of menopause delayed the future onset of Alzheimer's. It has been hypothesized that brief or long exposure to estrogen treatment affects Alzheimer's expression twenty to thirty years later by preventing the loss of precious neurons associated with hot flashes.

Whatever the case, the fact that estrogen can prevent, treat, or delay Alzheimer's is great news for any woman. My endeavor as a doctor of longevity is not to just extend the years but to also extend the quality. Research into Alzheimer's and estrogen is ongoing, and perhaps one day estrogen may be on the front line of Alzheimer's defense. Trial after trial has shown proof-positive results that with the supplementation of estrogen, there is a shining light in the prevention of Alzheimer's at the end of the tunnel.

The Estrogen Scare: Breast and Ovarian Cancer

Estrogen has been in the news quite a bit lately, and seems to have picked up some bad press. Some doctors and scientists speculate that estrogen causes such diseases as breast or ovarian cancer, and these claims are showing up in headlines and news stories across the nation. I am in a different camp of thinking altogether. What many of these news articles seem to omit is that the actual chances of women developing breast or ovarian cancer from the influence of estrogen replacement is relatively low. The risks are slim, but that hardly makes for an exciting news flash. Well, here is a news flash that maybe your doctor forgot to tell you—heart disease far surpasses breast cancer (about five to ten times) as far as what women are at risk for and the leading death from cancer is that of the lungs. The jury is still out on whether or not estrogen causes or spurs breast cancer, but really there is little proof that it does. Yet, the plain-as-day fact that estrogen protects the heart from disease and complications cannot be disputed. *Estrogen saves lives*, but unfortunately this truth is stained by the supposed threat of breast or ovarian cancer. Women see the word cancer and everything else fades to a blur in the background. I would like to put things back into perspective and again sharpen your focus—present-day data confirms that the paranoia over breast cancer is just that—paranoia.

In the previous segments in this chapter I illustrated through personal patient stories and clinical data the life saving benefits a woman can reap from taking estrogen supplementation. I showed you what estrogen can do, now I would like to talk about what estrogen does not or is not proven to do. I also want to help women understand that taking estrogen after breast cancer does not add fuel to the fire, and in many cases, estrogen has been shown to actually increase a breast cancer victim's chance of survival. If this is the case, then why the big scare, or where did doctors come up with the idea that estrogen causes breast cancer? Most likely from deductive reasoning: men have little estrogen, they also have little incidence of breast cancer or breast cancer cells containing biologically active estrogen receptors. These facts have seemed to support the hypothesis that estrogen causes breast cancer or at least spurs the growth of existing breast cancer.

This deductive reasoning has its place but studies have taken the rug out from under its feet, meaning they have proven it to be further from the truth. Some studies have actually shown that estrogen does not affect breast cancer, while other studies have illustrated a slight increase. To put this in perspective for you, I'll show you the rating scale for "relative risk." Everything we do either increases or decreases our risk for some disease or another. Eating a good diet will lower your risk, while smoking will shoot your risk to uncomfortable levels. In the rating scale, a number one is equal to no risk. This is important to understand since long-term use of estrogen in regard to breast cancer is a low risk of 1.4. This low relative risk hardly constitutes the harsh and unsubstantial claims newspapers and the six o'clock news are making about estrogen replacement therapy and breast cancer. I believe it to be faulty, one-sided reporting. I would like to show you the studies they're not citing, and let you make your own educated decision.

Over ten years ago, in 1987, researchers of the Cancer and Steroid Hormone Study observed women on estrogen therapy for twenty years or longer. They found no incidence of breast cancer, not even in women who had a positive family history of breast cancer. "Overall, the risk of breast cancer did not appear to increase appreciably with increasing ERT duration or latency, even for durations and latencies of 20 years or longer."

Another more recent study featured in the *American Journal of Preventive Medicine* showed an analysis from the NHANES I Epidemiology Follow-up Study that concluded there was no increased risk for breast cancer in women who used HRT. They found no statistically significant association between HRT and the development of breast cancer in the 5,761 women who participated in the study from 1971 to 1992.

It's also interesting that women who take oral contraceptives that contain two to four times higher doses of estrogen and progestin than found in hormone replacement therapy have no significant increase in breast cancer. In a 1985 issue of *Lancet*, a study concluded that women under the age of 45 did not experience an aggregate risk of breast cancer when taking a form of oral contraceptive.

Many women who have or had breast cancer are curious about whether or not they can partake in estrogen's many life-saving benefits. Many of their doctors would say no, and common practice is to avoid hormone replacement for woman who have or once had breast cancer. These women not only have suffered the trauma of breast cancer, but also now must face a life without the heart-healthy, bone-building, and mood-enhancing benefits of estrogen. Many studies are now showing that women who have survived breast cancer need not be deprived of estrogen's life-saving assistance. Many women who used hormone replacement or an oral contraceptive at the time of their breast cancer diagnosis showed improved survival rates over women who were not on either.

Bergkvist observed 261 women for nine years who were using estrogen at the time of their breast cancer diagnosis. He compared these women to 6,600 women who were also diagnosed with breast cancer but who were not using estrogen supplementation. His results were staggering. At the end of eight years, the group of women who used estrogen when diagnosed with cancer had forty percent fewer mortalities than the other group.

In a bolder study done by Dr. Philip DiSaia, an expert in gynecological cancer, forty-one women elected to take estrogen replacement therapy even after diagnosis of breast cancer. Their results were matched to eighty-two women who did not take estrogen. What Dr. DiSaia discovered is that women on or off estrogen showed no difference in survival or disease progression for periods of up to eleven years. I'm sure that is quite the oxymoron to the headlines you're used to seeing. What Dr. DiSaia didn't say is that the women who took estrogen, beyond not having trouble with their breast cancer, received the life-sustaining benefits characteristic of estrogen therapy.

With what is proven—estrogen maintains heart health, builds bone, perhaps (as far as initial studies are concerned) aids in cognition and emotional ailments common in the elderly, and eliminates the menopausal blues—it seems relevant to me that too many women are absent of its life altering effects. The doctor's oath is to "do no harm."

Doctor's feel they are upholding this oath by swaying their patients away from estrogen treatment because of the menacing threat of breast or ovarian cancer hovering in the future. I believe the threat is hardly menacing and what women should also be considering is the condition of their heart and the state of their bones.

Ovarian cancer is also rare. I saw recently an article in a March 2001 issue of *USA Today*, front page and center, headlines reading, "Estrogen-cancer link may be deadly." This, of course, is disturbing news to women taking estrogen or women deliberating on whether or not to take estrogen. It seems a rather open/shut case after headlines like that. But what women missed, if they failed to read on, is the citing of a recent study in the *Journal of the American Medical Association*, that "women who used ERT for less than a decade were no more likely to die of ovarian cancer than those who never used it." This hardly constitutes the harsh title the piece received. I always advise my patients to read between the lines and read carefully, and also to be wary of any large claims until you have a substantial amount of backing.

Estrogen *has* received a bad wrap when used in context with the subject of cancer. Yet, I wonder, have you heard recently that estrogen helps deter colon cancer. Colon cancer is more common in women than in men and is one of the leading causes of cancer incidence and deaths in women, a far more serious risk than breast cancer. Twenty studies have focused on estrogen's effect on colorectal cancer, and a majority of these studies have found a common ground in the suggestion that estrogen protects, with continued use, against the incidence of colon cancer. It's unknown how exactly, although hypotheses that it affects bile acid metabolism or promotes tumor suppressor activity have been discussed.

So, why do we as a public only get the negative side of the truth? It beats me. With estrogen being such a dynamic and essential hormone that offers both short and long-term benefits, it baffles me that women only know the possible risks but know nothing of its rudimental heart saving benefits. In a recent survey only 35 percent of women were aware of the connection between heart disease and menopause. (Wyeth-Ayerst Fourth Annual Menopause Report, 1996.) Sixty-five percent of women are without the proper knowledge that is imperative in making decisions about the second half of their lives. They are in the dark, waiting for the light to come in. I hope this book helps to throw open a door and let that light come in.

I understand that women with a history of breast cancer are still a contraindication, and in some cases, it would be wiser for them not to take part in an estrogen replacement program. But for women whose lives are severely impaired by estrogen deficiency, estrogen replacement is necessary. These questions and concerns should be approached with care and clear-minded understanding. When women approach me with apprehension, I lay all of the facts on the table. There is a *slight* risk of breast cancer, but there is a *dangerous* risk of heart disease and osteoporosis. A woman and her doctor must weigh her options, but make sure you, as the patient, are presented all of the options.

What Does this All Mean?

So many doctors have become lackadaisical in their prescribing care, and would rather be educated by big pharmaceutical companies, than educate themselves. It is so important to find a physician that is willing to be educated by their patient's needs. The reason I practice natural hormone replacement therapy today is that my patients demanded it. My patients motivated me to look further than what med school training offered and what pharmaceutical companies were pushing. Medicine is a dynamic field and if your doctor doesn't stay on his or her toes, the medical world will merely pass him or her by, leaving you without the most current care.

I'm advocating that every woman be on estrogen. Your doctor, of course, should weigh the options of your health, your heredity, and your needs before prescribing any hormone regimen. But I believe ultimately, your doctor should educate you and let *you* make this choice. Most women are eligible to reap the benefits of estrogen's longevity-enhancing therapy, but there are a few exceptions. Contraindications to taking estrogen include pregnancy, undiagnosed abnormal genital bleeding, acute thromboembolic disease, and a history of breast or endometrial carcinoma—although here, as I stated in the last segment, are some huge discrepancies. If you have any of the above problems, talk to you physician regarding methods of dealing with menopause and the aftermath of estrogen deficiency. This lifetime is the only one you've been granted. Like everything, it needs revising and reworking as the years pass. Estrogen happens to be the best tool to gear yourself up for the years to come. It builds bone, protects the heart, and might stop Alzheimer's in its tracks. It has been proven to save too many lives to let the minor risk of breast cancer cloud your vision. I urge you to open your eyes and reap the benefits.

Progesterone: Estrogen's Natural Side-Kick

Everyone in our office jokes about needing a progesterone pill when they're in a bad mood. It really does elevate your mood. Before, I felt like I was on pins and needles every day; now, although I still have the daily stresses, I feel better equipped to handle them.
—Antonia, 48

If I forget to take my progesterone for a couple of days all I do is cry and cry. It's amazing how it influences my outlook on life.
—Martha, 67

Progesterone finally captured the attention of physicians because of the success—and dangers—of the then-current form of estrogen replacement therapy. Estrogen replacement therapy was working miracles on menopause until the early 1970s, when researchers discovered that women on estrogen were demonstrating an increased incidence of uterine cancer. Estrogen, it seemed, came with a high price that most women were not willing to pay. Doctors and their patients shied away from estrogen, and women were again faced with the arduous task of balancing a normal life with the symptoms of menopause. Not only did they miss out on estrogen's amazing ability to wipe out menopausal symptoms, they also failed to benefit from estrogen's heart-healthy, bone-building, and mood-enhancing capacity.

By prescribing estrogen by itself, doctors were missing one of the fundamental tenets of total hormone replacement therapy: equilibrium. Hormones labor in concert to ensure the body's successful battle against age-related disease and the mind's ability to learn and retain information so that we can potentially live to a healthy, ripe age. This is the case of estrogen and progesterone. What the doctors and scientists overlooked in early hormone replacement therapy is how the female's body and sexuality are governed by two essential hormones, rather than just the obvious one, estrogen.

Estrogen left alone will become dominant, and it can become pretty heavy-handed with certain aspects of the female body. Absent of progesterone's balancing properties, estrogen can become an adversary of the uterus, causing such problems as uterine or endometrial cancer. When progesterone is added, the risk drops below the baseline levels. In a recent study, as well as past studies, the addition of progesterone has shown its uterine protective quality. Researchers found in a seven-year follow up study that hormone replacement therapy, in survivors of surgically treated endometrial cancer, did not cause a recurrence of that specific cancer. Dr. Disaia compared the outcome of two groups of women: 75 endometrial cancer survivors who opted for HRT and 75 women who were not treated with HRT. Dr. Disaia stated that the recurrence that was found in both groups—two in the HRT group (1%) and eleven in the group without (14%)—becomes a function of hidden, left behind tumor cells; not the result of newly introduced hormonal stimulation or new cancerous cell growth.

Progesterone prevents overstimulation of estrogen to receptor sites. It is vitally important to include progesterone in your menopausal regimen since it can either block or down regulate receptors, hindering estrogen from overstimulating estrogen-sensitive receptor sites in the breast and uterus.

But before I go any further with *why* you should be taking progesterone, you should understand progesterone's primary role as a gestational hormone. A woman's menstrual cycle is regulated through the action of two different hormones, estrogen and progesterone. Progesterone is produced in the corpus luteum, the adrenal glands, and in the placenta during pregnancy. During the first half of a woman's monthly cycle, estrogen levels rise as the follicles in the ovaries prepare for ovulation. Progesterone levels rise during the second half of the cycle, preparing the uterine lining to accept the fertilized egg. If the egg is not fertilized, progesterone levels, as well as estrogen levels, drop and menstruation takes place. Progesterone levels are also important in creating a nourishing environment for a healthy pregnancy. Without enough progesterone, a woman has a difficult time carrying a baby full term.

When a woman reaches her thirties, progesterone production begins to wane, and after menopause, the levels plummet to almost zero. Unfortunately, menopause was originally seen as an estrogen-only deficiency, and progesterone replacement therapy was considered unnecessary. When estrogen supplementation alone led to increased incidents of uterine cancer and an abrupt and massive decline in estrogen replacement therapy took place—progressive physicians finally went back to their drawing boards for more research on just how a woman's body functioned. What these doctors realized is that during and after menopause, progesterone works to promote feelings of vitality and healthiness. Later, a lack of progesterone can lead to some of the same problems as low levels of estrogen: osteoporosis, heart disease, a decrease in libido, and a significantly diminished quality of life.

What you will discover as you read this chapter is that progesterone should *never* be left out of your hormone regimen. Whether or not you have a uterus, studies and anecdotal patient accounts are shedding light on progesterone's role in a woman's health after natural menopause or induced menopause, such as what occurs after a hysterectomy. Studies on progesterone are relatively new compared to estrogen, and we are establishing more benefits as doctors and scientists examine this previously overlooked hormone more closely.

Ready to Get Off the Mood Swing?

One of my favorite comments from the ladies I treat with estrogen and progesterone is that they feel alive again. One lady in particular—we'll call her "Felicia"—used to call my practice quite often with complaint after complaint. She was always abrupt, rude, and never had a nice thing to say about herself or my staff. Finally, with much coercion, Felicia agreed to come in for an annual check-up. After asking a few questions and performing a standard exam, I determined that she go on natural progesterone and estrogen. Within a few weeks she called to thank me for taking away the huge weight she felt she had been lugging around for the last year. Her voice actually *sounded* lighter. She also sent flowers to my staff.

Progesterone has the amazing ability of acting as an antidepressant, mild tranquilizer, and natural painkiller. It can be a tremendous treatment for premenstrual syndrome (PMS), helping to eliminate symptoms like moodiness, irritability, bloating, and headaches. These symptoms are, in fact, often due to either erratic or abnormally low progesterone levels. Natural progesterone can also eliminate the symptoms of menopause, which can include emotional instability, headaches, and mood swings. As a matter of interest, for those women who are unable to take natural estrogen, natural progesterone can often be prescribed to treat many of the common symptoms of menopause and prevent some of the diseases associated with estrogen deficiency.

As I said earlier, around the time menopause hits, women are already experiencing some big revisions in their everyday story. Children are going away to college or getting married. Marriages change suddenly without the distraction of teenagers, and some couples find themselves adjusting to a new marital environment. Along with this, women are multitasked beings. They balance work with family and try to squeeze in a little time for themselves. Menopause can sometimes send this delicate balance reeling. Progesterone's natural calming effect can redirect the menopausal depression. Instead, it allows women to wake in the morning refreshed and revved for a new day.

A great example of this is the recent cross-sectional survey that examined the quality of life related to the physiological, somatic, and vasomotor effects in a group of women changing their progesterone therapy from medroxyprogesterone acetate (Provera) to a natural micronized progesterone. Their quality of life was assessed via telephone interviews using the Green Climacteric Scale and the Women's Health Questionnaire. All the women using the natural micronized progesterone related significantly greater relief from vasomotor symptoms, anxiety, and bouts of depression then they had felt when on the synthetic form. They reported improved perceptions of their vaginal bleeding patterns and menopausal symptoms. Eighty percent of the women were satisfied with the micronized progesterone and continued its use even after the study had finished.

As I'm sure you're well aware, the amount of sleep a person has influences a person's mood and health as well. One of menopause's most disrupting symptoms is sleep loss. I've had many patients complain they feel lethargic and apathetic during the day and anxious during the night. Progesterone has been shown to help eliminate sleeplessness, and with my own patients, it has worked wonders. In a 2001 study published in *Menopause*, twenty-one postmenopausal women were put in two different groups: the first on Premarin and Provera (the synthetic form), the second on Premarin and micronized progesterone (the natural form). After six months, researchers had collected enough research through sleep journal recordings and tests in sleep laboratories to assess results. The women in the second group, the natural progesterone group, attested to significantly improved sleep. There was no increase in the synthetic group. The women on natural progesterone slept better and felt better.

It's truly amazing how the body reacts to the sudden shift and decline of any hormone. Progesterone deficiency, as well as estrogen deficiency, can cause minor to major complications—ranging from moodiness to heart disease. When replenished, these possibilities decline significantly. Mood and energy are really only the icing on the cake when it comes to progesterone's awesome influence over the entire body. In combination with estrogen, progesterone can help eliminate the chance of heart disease; and as I said in the last chapter, that should be foremost concern.

Matters of the Heart

With heart disease statistics where they are, we as a medical society and you as a patient should review current orthodox medicine and make some serious revisions. Natural progesterone is rarely prescribed and in its stead women are taking Provera, its synthetic and less effective form. Unfortunately, Provera has proved to negate some of estrogen's heart healthy benefits, and in turn this has affected natural progesterone's reputation. So, let me clear up some misconceptions you may have encountered. First, Provera is not progesterone (I'll explain later in the Natural verses Synthetic section), although you may have been told by your health care provider that it is. Second, bio identical progesterone naturally supports estrogen to keep your heart working at youthful levels by positively affecting your lipids. One of the core reasons I'm writing this book is to dispel any myths or incongruities you may have come across in your pursuit for longevity. There are many out there, and your health balances on what source you choose to believe. This chapter, as well as the entire book, is based on grounded research to provide you with information and sources that are reputable.

Your heart was protected by estrogen and progesterone in your earlier days. With the menopausal initiation into second adulthood, progesterone, as well as estrogen, levels decline at a rapid pace. In their decreasing wake, your heart is no longer protected as it once was. I've already discussed how estrogen labors to keep the heart free of disease; but many people, doctors as well as patients, are unaware of how progesterone fits into the heart healthy equation. Because of Provera's known unsatisfactory effects, researchers have focused on how natural, bio-identical progesterone affects the heart. What they have ascertained is promising.

A person's lipid metabolism is usually a good determinant of heart health. It has already been proven that estrogen has a positive effect on cholesterol; but studies are now showing that progesterone may add an extra boost. In a German multi-center observational study, doctors monitored the efficacy and acceptance of two different regimens of postmenopausal hormone replacement therapies. The groups were separated by whether or not they took micronized progesterone continuously with natural estradiol or sequentially, days 16 through 25 of the monthly cycle. Both groups experienced considerable relief from menopausal symptoms. There was a reduction in cholesterol levels in both groups, but it was statistically significant in the group who was on continuous progesterone therapy. Also, within the latter group, lipoprotein levels were also reduced considerably.

The landmark study (I mentioned earlier in the Estrogen chapter), the *Postmenopausal Estrogen/ Progestin Interventions* or *PEPI Trials,* also stressed the importance of natural progesterone over its synthetic version in relation to the heart's health. 875 women, aged 45-64, were put on either estrogen alone taken daily, estrogen taken daily and synthetic progestin 12 days of the month, estrogen and synthetic progestin daily, or estrogen daily with natural progesterone 12 days of the month. Although it closely monitored these women for each regimens' effects on bone mass, endometrial modifications, or quality of life, the trial's primary focus was on the regimen's effects on the key risk factors for the heart. The results of this long-term study indicated that estrogen, and estrogen plus natural progesterone, provided the best results for lipid metabolism—increased HDL and lowered LDL levels. Fibrinogen levels, associated with blood clots, were decreased and there was not a significant gain in weight. The natural progesterone results on the heart exceeded those of the synthetic progestin, while offering the uterus protection from endometrial cancer. Women with a uterus who were given estrogen alone experienced a higher risk of abnormal cell growth of the endometrium, the women benefiting from the addition of progesterone did not.

Natural progesterone by no means replaces estrogen with its heart-healthy benefits, but studies are showing that it certainly does not hinder a woman toward a heart-healthier lifestyle. Studies, although done on primates, have yielded positive results and promise for women seeking longer and more vital lives. Reported in the journal *Nature Medicine*, researchers gave estradiol to a group of rhesus monkeys who had had their ovaries removed to induce menopause. Added to the estrogen was either the synthetic form of progesterone, Provera or natural progesterone. Four weeks later, after the monkeys had adjusted to their new hormones, they were injected with two chemicals that stimulate heart attacks. The monkeys supplemented with estrogen and Provera experienced severe constriction of the coronary arteries, which cut off blood supply to the heart, causing them to almost die had it not been for on hand emergency medicine. The monkeys receiving natural progesterone and estrogen, or estrogen alone, faired the best and recovered without the help of emergency drugs.

There should be great consideration and you should be selective when choosing the hormone replacement treatment you will use. As I have shown above, the synthetic form of progesterone, medroxyprogesterone acetate or Provera, has no protective features for the heart, and in fact it may do just the opposite. Some doctors believe that taking Provera may actually be worse than no therapy at all. And as far as the heart is concerned, I believe they are right. Natural progesterone, on the other hand, enhances estrogen's ability to stave off heart disease, and may have its own preventative techniques. Studies have shown that it enhances estrogen's capabilities by improving blood flow under the stress of exercise, helping to increase forced expiratory volume, and lowering pulmonary obstruction.

It's true estrogen *is* the essential ingredient for a healthy heart. Natural progesterone only enhances its ability. This is important to understand when so many doctors have become used to prescribing Provera as progesterone, and too many women are taking Provera and missing out on the rewards of estrogen. There are compounding pharmacies that formulate and dispense progesterone that matches exactly what your body produces at youthful levels. Natural, bio-identical progesterone has been overlooked far too long, and with heart disease at record highs and Provera studies illustrating its negative impact on the heart, it amazes me that doctors are still including it in their patients' regimens. I encourage you to take to heart the proven benefits of progesterone. If you're on estrogen and Provera, you may want to rethink exactly what you're trying to accomplish. You may be inhibiting the incidence of endometrial cancer (the main reason progesterone is used), but in the meantime increasing your chance of heart complications. Natural progesterone takes care of the cancer problem and positively affects estrogen's impact on the heart. With these facts in mind, I don't really see a choice. Let your doctor in on what the medical community is finding out. If he or she is not receptive, then perhaps it's time to search out a medical practitioner who is willing to listen. It's amazing, not only will you feel better, but your body will experience an overall sense of well-being and vitality throughout the rest of your years.

Bone Up

Progesterone takes estrogen's powers for bone care one step further—research has shown that rather than simply preventing bone loss, progesterone can stimulate bone-building osteoblasts. In other words, progesterone may help build new bone. As I said earlier, our bones are under constant construction, being made and unmade, which is how they stay strong and healthy. When the bone-breaking osteoclasts start far outpacing the bone-building osteoblasts—as they often do after menopause—our bones are left porous and susceptible to breakage.

Dr. John R. Lee, a long-time progesterone proponent and researcher, believes that osteoporosis may actually be a progesterone-deficiency disease. He observed how a healthy diet with calcium and vitamin D, combined with estrogen (Premarin) and natural progesterone affected one hundred postmenopausal women aged thirty-eight to eighty-three, all at risk for osteoporosis. On top of the supplementation of vitamins and hormones, the women were put on a strict diet and exercise regimen. He forbade them to smoke and to limit their alcohol consumption. After three years, he measured their bone density and found that in 63 women, not only was their boneloss halted, but the tests showed an increase in density—they were growing new bone to replace the old.

Other studies have shown how estrogen and progesterone affect both the bio-chemical markers of bone metabolism and bone mineral density. In a study featured in *Menopause*, researchers found that women supplemented with both estrogen and progesterone for a year had a significant bone mineral density increase in the lumbar spine and hipbone. They concluded that micronized (natural) HRT favorably decreased serum and urine markers of bone metabolism and prevented bone loss, while resulting in a slight increase of bone mineral density in the spine and hip.

Another study compared the differences of women's bone mineral density who took hormone replacement therapy to that of women who were not reaping its benefits. The researchers performed studies on paired bone biopsies obtained before and after two years of treatment. What they found is quite remarkable. Women on hormone replacement therapy displayed preservation of bone balance, while the women without it developed a more progressive negative balance. Women supplemented with HRT had no change in the appearance of their bones, while the women in the control group experienced a pronounced increase in erosion and osteoclastic erosion depth over the two-year period. The control group experienced an increase in resorption rate, while the HRT group demonstrated a significant reduction. The results of the tests illustrated that the hyperactivity of osteoclasts in the first phase of menopause can be quelled with a balanced hormone replacement regimen and thereby prevent osteoporosis.

Dr. Lee believes that perhaps natural progesterone is all that is needed to master the reflexes of menopause and later on the afflictions of osteoporosis. I personally, and respectfully, do not agree. If you'll notice, all the studies I cited above involve both hormones. It seems researchers understand the delicate and essential balance between estrogen and progesterone. It also seems that Dr. Lee feels it necessary to include estrogen in the hormone concoction he used in the study above. It has not yet been proven that progesterone has the same antioxidant qualities as estrogen, nor the same heart-healthy aspects of freeing up arteries and lowering LDL levels while elevating HDL levels. Estrogen is as important as progesterone to our aging clock, and one gear is useless without the other. Progesterone protects the uterus without any adverse effects of its own, and estrogen completes the tasks progesterone cannot.

There is one thing of absolute certainty—osteoporosis is a debilitating disease, and your risk of suffering from it can be greatly decreased through a balanced hormone replacement plan. That's why I urge you to find a doctor who is aware of the changing times, aware that menopause—treated with a balanced combination of estrogen and progesterone—is just the ticket to living a long and healthy life. I encourage you to "bone-up," and take that first step to longevity by ensuring you're on the right track with total hormone replacement with natural hormones.

Since I Don't Have a Uterus, My Doctor Says I Don't Need Progesterone...

One of the hardest aspects of being a doctor in the longevity field is the myths that are generated, as myths generally are, through people who should know better. I cannot count how many women have come to my office under the impression, through reading and through their healthcare practitioner, that they do not need progesterone in absence of their uterus. I've also had doctors argue with me over my supplementation of an unneeded hormone in patients who have undergone hysterectomies. They believe, as they were taught to believe, and as I once believed, that progesterone is solely an endometrial cancer inhibitor and if a woman doesn't have a uterus, she has no chance of experiencing endometrial cancer, and therefore does not need progesterone, right? This may be one of the most impractical and unreasonable myths regarding hormone replacement therapy. Ever since progesterone was approved as a preventive method against endometrial cancer, doctors cannot see beyond its stipulated use to appreciate its numerous benefits, *even* for patients who have undergone hysterectomies. It's common practice for doctors to overlook the essentialness of progesterone as non-applicable for women who have had their uteruses removed. There is nothing further from the truth. To those women who no longer have a uterus, I emphasize this: *your body now, as it has in the past, needs progesterone.*

The lack of progesterone can result in age related disease, just as readily as the lack of estrogen. Proper bone density, heart health, a satisfactory quality of life, and contentment all depend heavily on an optimal balance between estrogen and progesterone. Since studies have shown that natural progesterone halts the progression of osteoporosis by stimulating osteoblasts, which in turn stimulate bone growth and new bone formation, it is an absolute necessity for bone health in *all* women. It helps increase HDL and results in a greater reduction in cholesterol levels, and it naturally enhances the benefits of estrogen. There are really no reasons for your doctor not to prescribe you progesterone, yet offhand I can think of several reasons why you should be taking it. Uterine health should really follow heart, bone, and emotional well-being, as far as reasons why a doctor should prescribe progesterone. Heart disease and osteoporosis occurrence far outweigh the risk of endometrial cancer. These risks should be foremost in your doctor's mind. You should find a doctor with the right mindset, because to have the complete optimal hormone health, you need both hormones—they were the ingredients that, in part, designed the woman you are today.

Synthetic Vs. Natural

There is no doubt that estrogen and progesterone can help protect women against many of the diseases that accompany aging and that post-menopausal women on estrogen/progesterone replacement therapy tend to stay healthier. Yet, I'm sure many of you have heard alarming stories about estrogen causing cancer and other negative side effects (breast tenderness, rashes, acne, headaches, high blood pressure, loss of hair, and urinary tract infections) that may have left you wondering whether estrogen replacement and all its benefits are, in fact, too good to be true.

Unfortunately, most of the estrogen prescribed by doctors today is in the form of *synthetic* estrogen. Premarin, the most popular form of estrogen on the market today, is a good example. Because hormones are a natural substance, the FDA says their molecular structure cannot be patented. We've already mentioned what this means: no patent means no corner on the market for a drug company and no big payoffs from drug research. I'm sad to say that your health means big business to a lot of pharmaceutical companies. Because drug companies could not patent "natural," bio identical hormones, they turned to "synthetic" forms of these hormones. These hormones are structurally similar enough to human hormones to work with the body, but they are not identical to the structure of human hormones. Premarin, as a matter of fact, is made from the urine of pregnant mares and, therefore, is not an exact match for human estrogen.

A "natural" hormone's structure, as opposed to synthetic, is identical to the chemical structure of the hormone as produced in the human body. Natural estrogen does not depend on animal products like Premarin, whose primary estrogen is estrone, the estrogen linked with cancer. Prescription natural estrogen is usually comprised of estriol and estradiol, the less harmful estrogens. To me, it seems logical to replace an item with its identical match. You wouldn't substitute a Honda V6 for a Porsche engine—in the same respect, there is no rhyme or reason behind doctors replacing declining human estrogens with horse hormones. The female human body cannot comprehend Equilen, the horse estrogen, and does not have the facilities to convert it into any of the three human estrogens. Instead the liver converts it into equilenin—the metabolite some researchers believe is the source for cancer.

Similarly, doctors were on the right track when they determined that estrogen replacement needed the counterbalancing effects of its partner hormone, progesterone. However, instead of prescribing natural progesterone, they turned to what the pharmaceutical companies had to offer: synthetic progestin, like Provera. Provera is as unnatural as it gets. It was devised in a test tube in the late 1940's to look similar to progesterone, but it is definitely a distant relative. Progestins usually do more harm than good. In the *Physician's Desk Reference*, a good 60 percent of the text is devoted to contraindications and adverse reactions. Instead of nullifying the effects of menopause, Provera can cause breast cancer and in some cases also cause depression, weight gain, blood clots in the lungs or brain, water retention, and breast tenderness. Sounds worse than the actual effects of menopause. Despite the documentation on the benefits of natural progesterone, most women today are being prescribed synthetic progestins instead of natural progesterone. These synthetic progestins can cause the same problems and side effects as synthetic estrogens: bloating, headache, moodiness. The benefits from progesterone supplementation that I have described in this chapter are best achieved with natural progesterone rather than synthetic progestins. In fact, natural progesterone offers just as much cancer protection as synthetic progestins, better protection for the bone, and more improvement to mood.

In a specific study, Hargrove et al. compared natural progesterone with that of medroxyprogesterone acetate (Provera) in combination of estrogen therapy for menopausal women. They found that the women who were administered natural progesterone had a higher symptomatic improvement, an improved lipid profile, and did not suffer from breakthrough bleeding or hyperplasia. The women reported no side effects but rather an enhanced quality of life and sense of well-being and wished to remain on their treatment beyond the study confinements. However, two women in the Provera group requested to end their treatment due to severe side effects.

Other studies have shown that the use of medroxyprogesterone acetate or Provera, both synthetic progestins, can have some serious consequences to the female body above and beyond the side effects listed in the *Physicians Desk Reference*. Many women fear breast cancer and the impending possibility that hormone replacement therapy may be one of its causes. Many studies have concluded that *synthetic* hormone replacement therapy could be one of the root causes of breast cancer and that natural, bio identical hormone replacement is effective without these risks. Three studies in particular point the finger at Provera and medroxyprogesterone acetate as the culprits behind breast cancer emergence. Just recently, the *Journal of American Medical Association* (JAMA) concluded by assessing data gathered pertaining to 46,355 women and their incidence of breast cancers by recent occurrences, duration, and type of hormone use, that progestin (synthetic progesterone) added to estrogen increased breast cancer risk well beyond the associated risks of estrogen use alone. Another study in the *Journal of Clinical Endocrinology and Metabolism* illustrated the same results by evaluating 86 postmenopausal women who were categorized as: 1) estrogen alone; 2) estrogen + medroxyprogesterone acetate; or 3) no HRT at all. The outcome was nothing short of appalling. The addition of the synthetic progestin resulted in greater breast epithelial cell proliferation and density as compared to the estrogen alone or absence of HRT altogether. Furthermore, the proliferation occurred to the terminal duct-lobular unit of the breast, which happens to be the site where most breast cancers develop.

And finally, although it's not the last study concerning this subject, the *Journal of the National Cancer Institute* concluded an associated 10 percent higher risk of breast cancer for every five years a woman supplements with a synthetic progesterone.

When I prescribe estrogen and progesterone I prescribe natural, bio-identical hormones for several reasons. A recent article in the *New England Journal of Medicine* demonstrated that long-term use of synthetic estrogen does increase the formation of breast cancer. However, in Europe, most research trials have shown that *natural* estrogen, especially when taken in conjunction with *natural* progesterone, actually protects against breast cancer. In addition, using estriol, which is a weak estrogen, has been shown to lower the incidence of breast cancer. An article first published in the *Journal of the American Medical Association* indicated that there was enough presumptive and scientific evidence accumulated to prove that estriol is the safer estrogen, as it has been shown to actually decrease the incidence of breast cancer.

It's strange how we, as a knowledgeable and conscientious society, weigh our options—and our health. The Hargrove study above is a perfect example of the effects of natural hormones. They were safe and effective, and the women complied with their treatment—in fact, they wanted to continue even after the study ended. What angers me the most is that the Hargrove study took place in 1989, and more than a decade later, doctors are still prescribing synthetic hormones that are risky and unpleasant to their patients. Cancer, depression, and general malaise are sidestepped when *natural* hormones are employed. Premarin is natural to horses and there is nothing natural about Provera. Yet, these are the hormones most often prescribed. This is my advice, when you are handed a slip of paper with the prescription Premarin or Provera written on it, think twice about the goals of your health care practitioner and your own intent. Native or natural hormones are the key to a healthy longevity. They are an exact match to the hormones your body produces naturally and offer relief from not only bothersome menopausal symptoms, but also from the diseases that make living a long and prosperous life impossible. Natural hormones make it possible.

Aside from further decreasing any risk of cancer, it has been my experience that natural estrogen and progesterone simply leave women feeling better.

One of my patients, a 57-year-old woman which we'll call "Grace," complained that not only had she gained the ten pounds that often accompany menopause, but she also had less energy and was suffering from bladder leakage due to decreased muscle strength. It was difficult for her to exercise and when she did she would often feel worse afterward. Her doctor prescribed synthetic estrogen and progesterone but her symptoms worsened and she became depressed. Eventually she took herself off the synthetic hormones. Another physician tried another hormonal combination but this also made her feel worse and she quit that as well.

Finally, a mutual friend referred her to me. I started her on natural estrogen, progesterone, and testosterone. Within one month, she noticed vast improvement. The side effects she had experienced under her prior therapies were gone. She found she had improved strength and energy and saw a new person in herself. Her depression lifted, and she started her mornings with a desire to get up and go, whereas before she had not even wanted to go outside. And her husband was amazed at her revitalized interest in their sex life.

Another patient I worked with, a 49-year-old woman we'll call "Susan," who was going through menopause, was prescribed synthetic hormones that she felt did not agree with her body. In addition to feeling the hot flashes and mood swings associated with menopause, she felt that her health and energy had deteriorated as well. She no longer felt alive. Susan had asked her private physician to prescribe natural hormones. He merely stated that he had been using what he called "natural" hormones for the past 20 years and had had no complications.

Like many of my patients, her friends referred her to my office where we worked out a balanced prescription of natural hormones. After a matter of weeks, she called, excited to report the dramatic results. Susan stated that she was amazed by how quickly her menopausal symptoms had subsided and her overall feeling of well-being improved. She has been so excited about her results with natural hormones, she is eagerly telling her friends about this relatively new hormone replacement program.

I never advertise my practice because my patients both in their appearance and their enthusiasm spread the news like wild fire. Their new zeal for life makes them walking testaments to the kind of benefits a patient can reap from natural hormone replacement therapy. Both women and men alike, when supplementing their bodies with a complete hormone regimen, feel and look sexier, healthier, and vivacious. I've seen the pink color of youth restored to faces that looked pale and worn out by age and I've seen smiles return. The women above are only examples of the kind of benefits hormone replacement can offer.

The Challenge

Any woman who feels suspended in menopause limbo needs to know that there is more to life than feeling this way. Any women who wants to get the most out of the years to come now has the option and the capabilities to do just that. Do what thousands of women have already done—grasp life with both hands and mold it into the shape and length *you* want. You don't have to flounder through the pre-, ongoing, and after years of menopause. You can look and feel younger while you grow older. This isn't magic or some hidden fountain of youth. There is no mystery behind the benefits of natural hormone replacement therapy—you're only supplying your body with its natural tools to maintain a healthy long life. Medical advances in our society have extended the quantity of years; I'm working on extending the quality.

Natural progesterone and estrogen are out there. Don't do without their protection from heart disease, stroke, cancer, osteoporosis, and Alzheimer's disease. Let them improve your skin, mood, sex life, and self-image. Your next fifty to sixty years depend on it.

Testosterone:
Revitalize Every Aspect of Your Life!

What a piece of work is man.
—from William Shakespeare's *Hamlet*

I want to start this chapter with a story, because I believe stories paint pictures, and as we're well aware, a picture speaks a thousand words…

Once there was a man who had spent his life jumping hurdles and cunningly climbing social and political ladders until he found himself lunching in the higher echelons. His ambition had built him an economical empire and his decisions trickled down into many aspects of other people's lives; when he moved it seemed people held their breath so as not to disturb him. He held all the strings, and with one tug, could send a person's world toppling down. This sounds appealing to most men, this powerful resonance that engulfs a man's surroundings. But do you know this man also succumbed to a mid-life crisis? Can you imagine a man known for his perfect control, his lack of personal reflection at work, and his mapped out existence, suddenly confronted with an inability to control the inner environment of his own body? As with most men suffering andropause, he was ignorant to symptoms of his age-related hormone deficiency. He had never heard within and out of his social circles discussed anywhere that men suffered, like women, a sort of menopause.

Like many men, this hormone alteration suggested itself in the disguise of arrogance and aggression. The man lost his temper and exploded at the smallest inconveniences. These volatile tremors rippled throughout the company, unsettling the foundation he had worked so hard to build. His wife of twenty years felt she had wandered into the twilight zone whenever she entered a room he occupied. A frustrated silence engulfed their marriage. He began looking at younger girls, he bought more youthful clothing, and dyed his distinguished graying hair jet black; in effect, he tried to recreate himself.

You may be saying to yourself, "C'mon, this is so anecdotal, is this guy for real?" And I admit it *is* stereotypical, but stereotypes come into being for a reason. Hormonal declines affect every aspect of a person's health and well-being. We work to finally feel comfortable in our own bodies and after fifty years, we're assaulted with a whole new setting to adapt to. Some men stumble through this time, trying to make heads or tails of it, others seem to fly through it with no problem; some just suffer in silence. Testosterone levels are the answer to how well or how badly a man will encounter the transition into the rest of his adulthood. When a man with high levels of testosterone in his youth reaches fifty, his levels may drop, but not significantly enough that he may notice the change. Yet, more often than not, the blow, although gradual, *is* noticed. Unfortunately, for many men, this slow but sure decline hasn't been an issue of discussion, and like the example of the man above, ignorance does not always bring bliss.

I believe there is a general "agism" that infiltrates our culture, leaving men to grow old without proper body armor to defend against it. What if I were to say that you and I are expected, as odds would have it, to acquire cancer, heart disease, diabetes, Alzheimer's, osteoporosis, or if we're really "lucky" a general malaise. Why? Because we're getting older and weaker, and we're more susceptible to age-related disease. Basically, we're all expected to get old and suffer the consequences.

Yet, beyond this shortsighted agism are progressive doctors who do not view aging as a natural decay we're all subject to undergo, but rather, as a disease that can be treated and controlled. Some scientists and doctors view this approach as "wishful thinking." I, myself, believe any other alternative is a serious disservice to mankind. We *will* die eventually, but how and when we die is potentially our decision. I'm writing this book to give you the knowledge of that potential, and the information and the choices to take advantage of that potential and survive the rigors of aging.

I think this agism actually affects men more negatively than women. Because menopause is such a shocking and visibly life-altering event for women, the pursuit to eliminate the ailments has been a historical endeavor. Men, on the other hand, experience a gradual and seemingly more forgiving decline. The hormone that defines their male attributes dips little by little and therefore, the loss of youth is not as stripping as it is with women. Thus, a man's midlife crises has been underscored and ignored as purely a childish cling to a masculine ego. We see time and again the stereotype of midlife crises played out in the purchase of a new car or a sudden interest in younger styles and more youthful pastimes. As with all archetypal roles, this one is not without a source and I've seen many men stumble into this pitfall. This chapter is to educate you men who are salivating over that cherry-red corvette or finding more and more women attractive who are twenty to thirty years your junior. There is a remedy more cost efficient and less emotionally draining. I've seen testosterone work wonders for a man's ego and help marriages waning under sexual dysfunction and depression.

Unfortunately, many men are, as are many women, uneducated about andropause, or male menopause. The whole idea of men going through menopause and needing hormone replacement therapy is demasculinizing. Virility is a man's second nature and when hormonal changes occur, usually starting around the age of forty to forty-five (although some cases start as early as thirty or as late as sixty-five) men see a marked continual decline in abilities they once perceived to be as easy as breathing. Men find erections are not as frequent as they once were, sex is not as exciting because ejaculation is not as powerful, and the stamina and endurance they once experienced in both work and play has dropped as well. It seems that men, after forty-five, often have a hard time rising for any occasion. This is what is referred to as andropause, also known as male menopause or viropause. So why do most men not know anything about andropause? It has been only recently that andropause has received attention and recognition, but why the holdup? There are many reasons behind the stifling of its discovery along with many frames of mind that are still hindering its cure.

Because female menopause is so sudden and violent, ways to maneuver around its life-altering effects and health-diminishing aftermath have been under microscopic observation for decades. Women's bodies, in their hormonal revolutionary sense, are no longer medical anomalies. Doctors and scientists are well aware of the ramifications due to the absence of estrogen and progesterone. In the meantime, while men are scrutinizing over how women's bodies function beyond menopause, they have safely kept their focus from themselves and their own faulty faculties. Why? There are many reasons. Ignorance, pride, and plain surprise are a few that come to mind. I can't imagine my own grandfather, or even my father for that matter, pulling me aside to let me in on how life after fifty really feels. My grandfather never admitted defeat and this stubborn stoicism traveled from each generation to the next, as it does in most patriarchal families. Boys learn from their fathers to rise above their affliction and never give the slightest indication of weakness.

Slipping Into Lower Gear

The truth is, men are blasted with a reality check during their mid-forties. Their hormone levels drop and the erection that once greeted them in the mornings ceases, while their muscle definition fades and they notice they're getting a little flabby around the middle. "It's all a matter of aging," they're told and they settle grudgingly into old age.

Testosterone is truly a life source to the male body. Produced primarily in the testes by the specialized, Leydig cells (90 to 95 percent), along with a small amount produced in the adrenal glands, testosterone travels though the body via the bloodstream and binds to receptors on target tissues, which then issue the particular response needed. There are testosterone receptors all over the body, as well as important areas of the brain. Testosterone is the defining factor in a male's development. It's the flipped switch that, during puberty, sends boys reeling with the changes in their emotions and physical appearance. At this time, testosterone triggers the growth of pubic hair and facial hair, the deepening of the voice, and the general appearance of a more masculine shape.

Historically speaking, testosterone has been the subject of much scrutiny for centuries. The male's testicles and penis have, in various cultures, been symbols of fertility and virility. Fertility gods in some cultures were sculpted with the penis and testicles being the most prominent features. Other societies actually concocted love potions from the ground up testes of animals considered to be virile, like a bull.

What I find most interesting is testosterone's medical history, how forward doctors and scientists sought out the ability to master the power of testosterone into a supplemental form. As early as 1848, German professor Arnold Berthold shocked his community by transplanting young poultry testicles into the chests of two castrated roosters. He observed that his operation was a success in that it gave the roosters a sudden inclination to chase hens around the coop.

More than a decade later, in 1875, Charles-Edouard Brown Sequard, a French physiologist, stunned his colleagues by injecting himself with canine testicular fluid, his hypothesis being that the fluid would jumpstart his sex life and add zest and enthusiasm back into his work. He claimed the results were positive, that a true life-source had been added back into his aging frame. The scientific community first scoffed at his peculiar antics, but after several weeks of making the same bold claims of having enough youthful vigor to work longer hours and during those long hours, stand rather than sit, they took hesitant notice. Unfortunately for Dr. Brown-Sequard, the results could not be duplicated in other males. He was viewed as an old fool in search for the unattainable fountain of youth.

Perhaps Dr. Brown-Sequard was before his time, with his pioneering sense of science. He was on the right track, as were many cultures of antiquity, in that they understood that whatever was in the testes was vital to a boy's maturation into manhood and to his sexual appetite. It was not until 1931 that Adolf Friedrick Johann Butenandt, a German biochemist, isolated a few grains of the male hormone androsterone, a metabolically altered form of testosterone. Although changed from its source, it still produced a stimulatory effect on a cock's comb growth. Later, a Croation-born Swiss organic chemist, Leopold Ruzicka, synthesized androsterone and testosterone from cholesterol. His patented formula brought him riches and fame.

Both he and Butenandt received the Nobel Prize for their work in isolating and compounding testosterone.

From a historical standpoint, testosterone has been the mystical ingredient that emitted manly characteristics like strength and brawn. Cultures have tried various measures to capture this evasive male essence, but only succeeded as far as creating a placebo effect. From a medical standpoint, doctors and scientists have also been in the pursuit of this source. Equipped with science, they were able to isolate and later manufacture from cholesterol the core from which male characteristics are derived.

It was 1936 when Leopold Ruzicka discovered the chemical structure of testosterone. Since then, although we have the exact empirical formula, men who are suffering from low levels of testosterone usually go without it. Why? For a long time, endocrinologists believed testosterone levels were not affected by age. It has only been recently that an age-related testosterone decline has been detected and proven. One reason for this delay is that doctors were unable to get an accurate testosterone reading due to the natural ebbing rhythm testosterone displays during the day and even from season to season. Testosterone levels are funny, indeterminate subjects of study. A scientist cannot do a cross-sectional study (a study of comparison) of a group of young men against a group of older men and draw any sort of accurate conclusion of whether or not testosterone declines with age. Only a longitudinal study (a study carried out over a number of years) of the same group of men, can give a more precise idea of how testosterone declines.

Another reason endocrinologists did not believe testosterone took a dip after forty-five is because they measured the wrong type of testosterone—measuring the total amount of testosterone rather than focusing on the free testosterone. Much of a man's testosterone is tied up or bound to a protein called sex hormone-binding globulin. Once bound to SHBG, the testosterone is no longer obtainable to the rest of the body. There is only a small amount of bioavailable or free testosterone accessible to the body, about four percent. Research has shown that free testosterone becomes more bound with age, leaving readily available levels of testosterone low, while total testosterone levels are normal. This is where one of the biggest hang-ups has occurred and where symptoms of aging were not tied to a testosterone decline. It was not until doctors and scientists honed in on the bioavailable testosterone did they realize there was a definite drop.

So, not only is science relatively new as far as testosterone replacement is concerned, but society as a whole is ignorant to the benefits of testosterone and the symptoms involved with its decline. In a 1998 survey sponsored by the ALZA Corporation, over one thousand men were asked questions pertaining to their knowledge of testosterone and hormone replacement therapy. The outcome of the questionnaire revealed that 68 percent of men could not name one single symptom of low levels of testosterone, only 15 percent named decreased sex drive, 6 percent cited fatigue, and 3 percent came up with less lean muscle mass. Only one percent named loss in bone density. More than *half* had never heard of hormone replacement therapy, while only a quarter had, and attributed it to a female-only procedure. Only a small percentage of men had ever heard of hormone replacement for males.

This is why this chapter is extremely important. I think its time to come out of the dark ages and take control. The truth of the matter is that testosterone levels do decline. They actually decline in two separate ways. There are two life-altering processes conveniently wrapped up into the terms, primary and secondary hypogonadism. With either of these declines come a slew of complications ranging from a lack of sexual desire to a serious risk of heart disease. There are many contributing factors in testosterone's switching into lower gear. One is that the testosterone-producing Leydig cells, located in the testes, reduce in number over time and cannot produce testosterone at youthful levels, known as primary hypogonadism. Another root of testosterone's decline takes place in the chain of information, which first emerges in the pituitary gland, then prompts the release of luteinizing hormone-releasing hormone, which in turn stimulates the testes to make and drive out testosterone. It's a step by step process that age interrupts, and as a man grows older the luteinizing hormone-releasing hormone become less sensitive to the pituitary's signals and testosterone production begins to wane. This last form is termed secondary hypogonadism. Above and beyond hypogonadism, men experience an abnormal displacement of estrogen. This estrogen imbalance is more likely the chief cause of andropause and also its most hushed source. Men don't want to know their testosterone will take on a more girlish figure and that the results, at best, will be uncomfortable, or at worst, deadly.

The Estrogen Dilemma?

It's always interesting to watch the expression on a male patient's face when I mention his estrogen levels. It can only be described as a shocked pause of disbelief. I sometimes expect them to turn around to see if I'm talking to someone else in the room. Men and women are not black and white, and although we may feel comfortable saying one is from Mars, the other from Venus, it all boils down to our biological truths: men and women are affected by the same hormones, although at differing degrees.

Believe it or not, estrogen is actually produced by the one thing in the body that is absolutely male—testosterone. An enzyme called aromatase takes testosterone and molds it into estradiol, which is easy since it takes a closer look to distinguish the differences in their two chemical structures. As men age, aromatase is produced in larger amounts, causing larger amounts of testosterone to be converted into estrogen. Suddenly the balance, or ratio, is grossly tipped to estrogen's side, which in turn negates testosterone's beneficial effects on the heart, mind, and sex drive. Because of their similarities in structure, estradiol has no problem masquerading as testosterone and binding to testosterone's receptor sites. Once locked onto a cell membrane, estrogen bars serum testosterone from its rightful place, and therefore stops it from sending off healthy and productive hormonal signals. Some of my patients have exceptional levels of bioavailable testosterone but still harbor the ailments of a hypogonadal victim. This is the by-product of excess estrogen, which strips testosterone of its cellular receptor sites, leaving it void of its purpose. When it's deterred from receptor sites in the brain, the nerves, the muscles and genitals—sexual function and desire plummet. It's also a surplus of estrogen that tricks the mind into thinking that there is an overflow of testosterone, and therefore the hypothalamus signals to the pituitary to stop the process for testosterone production.

For years this oxymoron baffled doctors and scientists. Men with high free testosterone levels were complaining of dull sex drives and depression. Testosterone treatment proved to be worthless and these men watched as their sex lives went westward. It wasn't until recently that the culprit, estradiol, was located and understood. I don't want you to think that estradiol is solely an adversary to the male body. It has been shown to positively effect the masculine brain, and may also have it's own salvaging effects on the bones. Too little estrogen has an impotence effect, just as it does when it is in excess. If it's at its optimal levels, estrogen can play a positive part in our masculinity. In youth, a male's estradiol pragmatically turned off testosterone's powerful cell-stimulating effects; essentially it worked to keep testosterone in check and his body balanced and well tuned. However, when it surpasses those levels, it can potentially upset the entire chemistry of a male body. It keeps testosterone's "on" switch perpetually off, and forcefully takes its place.

There are many things that can factor into why estrogen is made in such abundance as a man gets older. Age bumps up aromatase activity a notch, changes how the liver functions, may cause a zinc deficiency, or obesity, or can be influenced by an alcohol intake, or by prescription drugs; all these may contribute to an estrogen dominance. I talked about aromatase activity above, but I also would like to explain some of the other key players in estrogen's break down of the male body.

The liver: Our liver is like the body's sieve. It aids in the expulsion of unneeded chemicals, hormones, drugs, and metabolic waste products from the body. In the male body, if working properly, it rids it of excess estrogen. With the consumption of alcohol and other factors, the liver undergoes a transformation and is no longer able to sift estrogen out of the body.

Alcohol Use: Alcohol has a queer effect on estrogen. While it's depressing some of our other systems, it's stimulating an increase in estrogen levels. Not only that, as stated above, it inhibits the liver's elimination of estrogen from the body, while decreasing zinc levels.

Zinc: Zinc is a mineral that puts the reins on aromatase activity and dampens estrogen's ability to grow too big for its britches. Unfortunately, in my opinion, the importance of zinc is downplayed and many people go without a proper supplemented amount in their diet. On top of that, alcohol and prescription drugs lower zinc's levels. Zinc and the pituitary have a close bond—without zinc, the pituitary has a more difficult time sending signals to the testes to produce testosterone. Although zinc is a definite ally to testosterone, it also seems that testosterone helps maintain zinc levels in bodily tissues.

Obesity: Fat cells contain aromatase. As we grow older, we also grow bigger around the belly. This complacency toward gaining weight as being just another fact of life contributes to testosterone levels going down and estrogen levels going up. As the fat cells accumulate, aromatase enzymes convert testosterone to estrogen.

Prescription Drugs: Many people in America are taking diuretics (water pills) to combat high blood pressure. Diuretics wash the all-important zinc from the body and therefore increase the chance of an estrogen power play. Although diuretics are used to keep blood pressure from skyrocketing, it's indirect cause of high estrogen levels actually do more harm to the heart in the long run.

Strike Two, Testosterone's Other Foe

Excess estrogen can also create an influx of sex hormone-binding globulin (SHBG). As I explained before, most of the testosterone is tied up in these proteins, leaving men with about four to seven percent of free, usable testosterone. When these added proteins, which are consuming more and more of our free testosterone, couple with estradiol, which is attaching to testosterone's cellular receptor sites, men experience a rough and downward journey into andropause.

This is all relatively new information. Doctors and scientists are just barely rummaging around in the male endocrine system (really within the last several decades) and it seems to have presented them with several mysteries that are difficult to untangle. I've read countless articles, participated in a myriad of discussions, and I've found that many of us have different hypotheses of not only why andropause occurs, but also of ideas on how to cure it and its many contributing factors. It will be interesting to see how it all pans out.

How do we achieve optimal levels of testosterone in the mean time? Through research and trial and error, we've discovered ways to inhibit estrogen dominance, thereby also lowering the chance of SHBG overproduction. Since the aromatase enzyme increases with age, and testosterone supplementation gives aromatization more opportunity to occur, research has been directed toward ways to limit this action from taking place. There are certain prescriptions, like Arimidex, which are relatively free of side effects and effectively prevent testosterone and other hormones from converting into estrogen. There are also natural supplements that seem to accomplish the same thing. Naturally occurring products, like the powerful antioxidant flavanoid chrysin, inhibits estrogen by suppressing the aromatase enzyme. Another herb that seems to free up testosterone to do its hormonal duty is nettle. European researchers have found that constituents of nettle actually bind to SHBG in place of testosterone, thus leaving testosterone free to settle into the receptor sites needed for sexual and cognitive function. It basically displaces androgens from the sex hormone-binding globulins. These are just a few of the beneficial ways to treat the aromatization that seems to creep up on men as the years pass by.

It's amazing that almost forty years ago we put a man on the moon, that we can now split the atom, that we can exchange a heart for one that is artificial and provide a man a way to live beyond a heart that wants to die. We have made medical and technological leaps and bounds, yet we still are mystified by the inner workings of male biology. We're finding one obstacle after another, and the sad truth is, we've had a late start. That is why I hope every man reads this chapter, so that as his bodily systems retire and he begins to feel "old" he'll, first of all know he's not alone, and second, he'll seek help. Make sure that when you do, you find a physician willing to talk about testosterone replacement and a physician willing to check all your levels, including your estrogen levels. It's those estrogen levels that will really prove to make or break a man as he ages.

The Ultimate Aphrodisiac

We now know that 60 percent of all men by the age of sixty-five have low levels of testosterone. We also know that testosterone levels are directly linked to a man's sex drive. It is not a coincidence that when boys go through puberty their sexual awareness soars. Nor, is it a chance happening that this awareness dulls into a frustrated indifference during a man's mid-forties to early fifties. The sexual dexterity a man was once proud of becomes a sporadic and less passionate visitor. For men with already low levels of testosterone, the tapering off is felt acutely. A fair amount of my male patients have come to me after suffering in silence for years (usually at the goading of a dissatisfied wife or lover). They shuffle around their symptoms, have a hard time looking me in the eye, and wait for me to make the educated guess—their sex drive is at its all time low. You can't imagine the disdain on their face when I tell them this is normal, but of course this dissipates when I let them in on the best kept secret—there *is* a cure.

I remember, specifically, a patient—we'll call him "Sean"—who was seventy-eight when he finally came to visit me. What prompted his visit is a great story, which sadly begins with a tragedy. Sean had lost his wife to cancer and after two years had met and married an attractive woman twenty years his junior, whose company he enjoyed immensely. Although they were compatible in most aspects of their companionship, he felt he lacked the passion and adventure she had under the covers. He had become accustomed to the infrequent lovemaking he and his wife shared during the last years of their marriage, and this new pressure made him frustrated and embarrassed at his lack of sexual appetite. He felt rusty and awkward. His friends and general practitioner basically advised him to take it easy, that he was no longer expected to perform sexual acrobatics, and that this was what old age was all about. Sean felt guilty that he couldn't keep up with his young wife and this guilt began to effect their relationship.

Luckily, he ran into an old college buddy of his, and a current patient of mine. Over coffee they began to compare notes about their social lives and found that they had a few similarities—they were both married to younger women. Yet, his friend spoke of the experience with excitement and optimism. His friend shared his secret, and Sean soon made an appointment to visit me.

Sean's problem was not hard to decipher, his testosterone levels were quite low. We designed the perfect dose to meet his needs and after two months, Sean and his wife are experiencing an exciting life beyond, and in spite of, what society calls "old age." He told me it felt like someone rewound his life a full twenty years and pushed play again. His wife also wrote me a letter, thanking me for the freshness that "whatever I did" added to their relationship. "He's much more playful and alive now. We've grown closer over the last three months than I've ever been to any man." Sometimes I chuckle to myself, thinking that perhaps one day she'll be straining to keep up with him.

This is a personal story of how testosterone supplementation can enhance the quality of a man's sex life. There are many documented studies that illustrate the same positive outcomes. In 1993, Fran Kaiser, M.D., of St. Louis University Medical School, released results of a study involving twelve men over the age of seventy, six of whom were given injections of testosterone, while the other six received a placebo. The men who received the testosterone reported a boost in their sex drive and function along with an improvement in their energy. Dr. Kaiser accounted that the men had not only gained weight and muscle mass, but also experienced lower cholesterol levels and their bones became stronger.

Most men have a hard time owning up to sexual dysfunction. Their sex lives are one of the aspects that defines them, and when that aspect declines or stops, many undergo an identity crises—thus the drastic changes in clothing style, hairstyle, or attitude. Although, here, I would like to insert a little cautionary disclaimer: since sexuality is such a dynamic part of our character, there are certain facets that affect sexuality that testosterone cannot help with. Testosterone cannot help a man that suffers from a sexual psychosis, but possibly other medications and emotional counseling can; this also goes for men who suffer from clinical depression. For other cases, such as the usual gradual decline of testosterone, supplementation is just the spice to heat up a man's sex life, in more than on way. Testosterone has been illustrated in some studies to affect the nerves and skeletal muscles involved in erections. We're still unsure of the exact workings, but its obvious in studies and in the testimonies of my patients that testosterone can work out the kinks and get the gears working properly again. Not only that, but testosterone can rev up a sluggish and listless sex drive. It increases sensation, improves orgasm, and overall satisfaction. I guarantee you'll feel a difference. A low testosterone level not only creates mechanical problems, it can also affect an overall outlook on sex. So many of my patients, when they first come to see me, say they "just don't feel like it" or they're "too tired." After a few months of testosterone supplementation, these same men feel a sudden zest in their sex lives and their wives or lovers are suddenly surprised with the lack of sleep they get at night. Believe me, no one's complaining.

In a Slump?

Our emotional stance in life can directly influence every action or reaction we have, whether it be in bed or in other areas or life. Depression breaks down a man's assurance and I've seen in more than one instance, depression can change a man totally.

How men deal with their emotions usually diverges drastically from how women express themselves. Women can usually articulate their emotions, albeit through crying or "talking." Because women have a socially accepted form of release, they are usually emotionally healthier creatures. In contrast, what I've noticed in my male patients is how they cope with their midlife transition. Many display anger and irritability while trying to adapt themselves to life after forty-five. This is understandable—as a man sees his life change and certain innate functions become more strained and less frequent, he becomes aggravated about this sudden lack of control within his own life. As a result, marriages suffer, as well as family and work, and unfortunately men are not versed in this natural phase in their life, so they do not recognize the signs and therefore cannot seek out the proper channels to receive help.

Sexual function, as I spoke about before, influences a man's mood, and his mood can impact his ability to have and maintain an erection. It's a two-way street that affects a significant amount of aging men.

What I have noticed in my practice is that many of these men have low-normal levels of testosterone. With the proper dosage, these men come alive again in both their home and in their office. They're more aggressive, not in the negative way some critics would like to persuade, but rather, their aggression motivates their success within their career and their desire to maintain a happy and prosperous personal life.

Many studies reinforce testosterone's reputation as being the feel good hormone that pulls men out of the mid-life rut. Hypogonadism or even just low-normal levels of testosterone impairs a man's sexual ability and also seems to fog his perception of life. Testosterone levels below 2.0 to 4.5 microgram per liter is linked to both sexual dysfunction and despondency. Whether administered intramuscularly, transdermally, or orally, testosterone has shown itself to be a strong ally to a man's ego and sex drive. It not only increases a man's mood but it puts him *in* the mood.

In today's culture, we have pill after pill designed to undermine depression. Depression is one of America's most deadly disorders and seems to have no preference for age or sex, although, statistically, the rate of suicide for men forty-five to sixty-four is three times higher than the rate of women of the same age. For men over sixty-five, the rate jumps to nearly seven times higher. Being a man on the cusp of these statistics, I find the numbers startling and sobering. I think there are many reasons women fare better than men. Perhaps one of those reasons is that women are supplemented with the vital hormones their bodies stop making naturally. Many women do not go without estrogen and progesterone, the feel-good hormones that buffer women against the effects of daily stress or the onset of depression.

One of my patients, fifty years of age—we'll call him "Greg"—was referred to my clinic by his psychiatrist. After almost a year of sampling different antidepressants and finding no positive results, Greg was directed to my office to have a complete hormone deficiency evaluation.

He confided in me that the antidepressants were killing his sex drive, and that in the heat of the moment, he couldn't get or maintain an erection. He expressed that it was increasingly hard to concentrate at work and he had a hard time attending to assignments, which were formerly awarded to him for his ability to be quick and concise. The thought of exercise overwhelmed him. By the time he got home from work at night, he was exhausted from just thinking of all the things he needed to accomplish.

I put Greg on a hormone regimen, including testosterone, designed to fit his particular needs. Within one month, Greg did an about face. His antidepressants no longer had ill effects on his sex life. After an additional month, he again had the fire and drive to accomplish assignments at work. His relationship with his wife got the boost it needed both sexually and emotionally. The combination of hormone replacement therapy and antidepressants has completely turned his life around. His mental clarity sharpened and he's full of the get-up-and-go and optimism he thought he had lost along with his thirties.

Greg almost fell victim to what so many people refer to as the inevitable fate—aging. What Greg didn't realize is that fifty is still a prime age, and so is sixty, and seventy. There's no reason a person needs to wind down into old age prematurely. There's actually no reason for a person to wind down at all. Most of my patients, before coming to me, have been on the verge of "giving up the ghost," so to speak. Their apathy and resignation dimmed their vision to the possibility of an active life beyond fifty-five. This apathy is truly a person's worst enemy, because it is this kind of indifference that gives age momentum and potency, allowing it to have the final say.

How About Changing That Spare Tire

When someone says the word "testosterone," an image usually jumps to mind of something rugged, something rough, something aggressive, something that makes men, men. When someone says the word "steroid," suddenly the image changes to something illegal, something that has darkened the reputation of sportsmanship, something that can seriously impede the health of its user. Unfortunately, it's these last few images that have put a damper on testosterone's good name. Anabolic steroids derived from testosterone, sold under names like Nandrolone and Oxandrolone, were employed by athletes in the 1950s to enhance their physical performance. These anabolic steroids increased muscle bulk and shortened the recovery time needed for muscles after a strenuous workout. There are people out there who misuse testosterone for its muscle-enhancing and fat-trimming benefits. These people are not experiencing a testosterone deficiency, but through professional sports or bodybuilding motivation, feel its necessary to add that extra push. Unfortunately, that extra push in people not deficient can sometimes cause some pretty serious consequences. Young athletes abusing anabolic steroids are in danger of sterility, liver damage, cancer, or even death.

Using anabolic steroids gained sour recognition in 1988 when Canadian sprinter Ben Johnson was stripped of his gold medal after tests indicated steroid use. Unfortunately, steroid pushing by high school and college coaches all over the world went unknown. Then on February 27, 1991, anabolic steroids were placed on the controlled drugs list. The U.S. Olympic committee banned the use of all male hormones by athletes.

As a doctor who prescribes testosterone, I am careful of who I do and do not prescribe testosterone to. There are many times I have to turn men away who are in their mid-thirties, muscle-bound and desperate to augment what they already have. It's my job, as a physician, to be responsible with testosterone's awesome capacity to rebuild a man to what he was in his youthful prime and not the other way around. As a hormone replacement doctor, I replace hormones back to optimal levels as they decline, not supplement hormones when there is no call or need for them. Therefore, I have put an age limit on my patients. It's a rare case when I prescribe hormones to men or women under the age of forty, forty years old being my standard starting age. Some of the cases where I will make an exception include, for women, early surgery-induced menopause, and for men, such debilitating problems as early hypogonadism.

As a healthy man grows older he begins to grow around the middle. When we look at black and white pictures of our fathers in their youths and compare them to our fathers now, we will most likely notice a marked difference. Men usually fall victim to central or visceral obesity, known also as the "pot belly," the "beer gut," or the "spare tire." Most men joke about their growing stomach, but there is nothing funny about the risks associated with adding on the inches. This spare tire increases a man's risk of cardiovascular disease or type II diabetes. As men take on the battle of the bulge, muscle melts into fat and exercise seems, with each passing year, to become a feat of will power as well as ability. Most of my male patients come to me with jokes about their belly; they use humor to deal with the changing shape of their body. It's humbling to observe your own body soften over time.

I remember one of my patients who had tried everything, from stepping up his workout regimen to virtually starving himself. The spare tire was absolutely stubborn to all his efforts. One day, Frank happened upon an advertisement of a lecture I was giving and decided to give it a listen. A few days after the lecture, he made an appointment with my office, where we determined his testosterone levels were fairly low. I prescribed him testosterone cream and after several months Frank's testosterone levels were restored to optimal levels. His belly did a disappearing act, and his body as a whole became harder and more defined. He told me he didn't remember looking and feeling this good even when he was thirty.

In 1996 this kind of testimonial was put to the test and reported in the *New England Journal of Medicine*. Researchers randomly assigned forty-three men to four different groups:

1. the placebo with no exercise group.
2. the testosterone with no exercise group.
3. the placebo with exercise group.
4. the testosterone with exercise group.

The men were administered either testosterone or a placebo weekly for ten weeks. The men in the exercise group lifted weights three times a week. What they found at the end of ten weeks was that both groups of men taking testosterone had significantly bigger triceps and quadriceps than the men in the placebo groups. Even without exercise, testosterone was able to increase muscle bulk, but of course the men in the testosterone plus exercise group faired the best as far as fat-free muscle mass and strength went.

Other studies have confirmed testosterone's benefit in older hypogonadal men. After oral or intramuscular testosterone treatment, elderly hypogonadal men experienced increased lean muscle mass, along with increased leg and upper body strength.

Study after study confirms testosterone's powerful influence over the masculine figure. With its decline men put on the pounds and sluggishly haul it around. But here's the good news, there is no reason to settle into your oversized body and there is no reason to accept your spare tire. Your fat-to-muscle ratio increases because your testosterone decreases. Your energy levels slacken, your mood levels dwindle, and you begin a life of fewer possibilities. Hormone replacement therapy opens up that world of possibilities. With the supplementation of testosterone, a man has the stamina to be a husband, father, professional, and sportsman late into his eighties. It's amazing what a small amount of testosterone will do for a man's self image and strength.

Out with the Old, In with the New

Our bodies are houses of very delicate architecture. As I have explained before, each facet depends upon another, whether it be one single cell or the entire skeleton. Like in a house, if a beam receives too much wear and tear or the foundation gives a little, each modification changes the entire appearance and health of the structure. Our bodies, from the moment we are born to the moment of our passing, are bombarded by internal and external erosion. Without the proper maintenance of our muscles or the continual healthy and balanced remodeling of our bones, our bodies will collapse in slow motion. Some of the most powerful tools in keeping the body in prime shape are hormones. Our bodies are sensitive to the slightest hormonal shifts. As each hormone dips or ebbs, our bodies react accordingly, and when a hormone *really* dips, our bodies counter with their own decline. Optimal levels of hormones are the keys to a body's ability to be built to last. As we get older, "built to last" usually means taking matters into one's own hands.

As men pass through andropause they encounter the risk of osteoporosis. Most men attribute this debilitating disease to a female frailty, but the truth of the matter is men become just as susceptible when their testosterone levels sink below normal. Because the life span in men is increasing, and as the more health conscious baby boomers add years to their lives, the bone fractures in men are expected to double by 2025. Muscles support bone while bone supports the body, and the older we get, both the insulating muscles and the bones they wrap around get weaker and weaker.

Sex hormones have always been involved in the development of our bones, starting with the period when we were still cradled in our mother's womb. Later, they influenced the linear growth spurt we experienced in our puberty years. While we were thinking of raging hormones as Mother Nature's curse, they were actually stretching our adolescent frames into the masculine or feminine bodies we now have as adults. But as we pass through our late forties into our early fifties, the mechanisms that maintain bone growth by the method of "out with the old, in with the new," become muddled. Without testosterone, the remodeling process picks up the pace, and there is a distinct loss of bone mass; osteoclasts (the old bone removal crew) leave deeper and closely spaced crevices in the bone, and the propensity for fractures escalates. Once a fracture occurs, the quality of life slips and we're forced to live life more carefully. Interestingly, a man who suffers a hip fracture is more likely than a woman to succumb to death soon after the event. In a presentation, Wehren and colleagues illustrated that even with the proper adjustments for preoperative differences in health status, depression, other diseases, operative complications, and other factors, men still had a two-fold chance of mortality due to complications from a hip fracture.

Sex hormones have been the focus of the bone debate, and over time, researchers have found they directly influence and regulate the birth and life span of osteoclasts and osteoblasts. The relationship between osteoclasts and osteoblasts is a delicate one, and any upset will cause havoc on our skeletal system. Both estrogen and testosterone foster a compatible and symbiotic liaison between the two juxtaposed cellular structures of osteoblasts and osteoclasts. The rate of osteoclast and osteoblast genesis and apoptosis relates to the health and longevity of bone tissue. Testosterone has been shown to help this process remain equalized.

Studies have shown that hypogonadal men experience vertebral and cortical bone loss, with reduced cortical, vertebral, and trabecular bone densities. They have an increased risk of hip fracture, and without testosterone, it seems, their bones whittle away. History has shown us as early as 1948 that testosterone administration helps reduce calcium excretion. With years of trying to understand testosterone's impact on the bone, researchers have come to the conclusion that six to eight months of supplementation increase the spinal bone mineral density in all elderly hypogonadal osteopenic men, mean age

61 years. Almost fifty years later, in 1996 researchers discovered that male test subjects who were administered testosterone not only had an increase of bone density at the spine of 5 percent, but also the trabecular bone mineral density increased a whopping 14 percent. It goes to show how science unravels the mystery of the endocrine system layer by layer.

I recommend above and beyond a dedicated diet of calcium and vitamin D, added to a good exercise regimen, that my patients also achieve optimal results by supplementing their body with something that deters bone loss. Estrogen eliminates gross percentages of bone loss in women, and preliminary studies have shown that testosterone administration accomplishes the same results in men.

The idea of testosterone preventing osteoporosis is a relatively new one. Many scientists have believed that aromatized testosterone (testosterone converted to estrogen) is the only kind that can positively affect bones. New research shows that men with complete androgen insensitivity due to mutations in the androgen receptor gene on the X-chromosome have decreased bone mineral density in spite of the fact that their estrogen levels are high. This has also been the case in women who suffer from androgen insensitivity syndrome. Although they comply well with their estrogen therapy, they experience a decrease in their bone mass. In rodents, nonaromatizable androgens, as well as other androgens, have identical effects as estrogen on the activity, as well as the birth and death of the specialized bone cells, osteoblasts and osteoclasts, in both in vitro or in vivo studies. Androgens have also proved to inhibit bone loss in ovariectomized rodents.

Male osteoporosis is just barely being recognized. Scientists and doctors are finding they need to revamp the measuring systems they have used on women, since male and female bodies are so different. Low bone mineral densities in women are not the same in men. Although women suffer more severely from osteoporosis, we are finding more cases of men who have passed through andropause, experiencing losses of bone mass. I attribute this to the decrease in testosterone and the loss of muscle mass as a result. Men have a decrease in energy and find it next to impossible to expend what they do have at the gym. Without the resistance that lifting weights and certain sports put on the bone, which causes the bone to grow in mass and strength, bones deteriorate. The lack of testosterone is a double-edged sword. If you don't have enough testosterone your bones suffer the consequences; at the same time, you don't have enough energy to physically, through sports, alter the downward spiral your bones experience after fifty. We have discovered that testosterone works its own miracles on the bone. It arrests the overzealous osteoclast activity and fosters a better working relationship between it and its close cousin, the osteoblast. When a man comes to me and complains he has lost an inch or two, the first thing I do is set him up for testosterone lab testing. It never fails that his testosterone levels are below normal. I've personally witnessed how testosterone, in many of my own patients, has positively altered a faltering skeletal structure. I've seen increased energy levels, increase lean muscle mass, and bone mineral densities rise in number. Testosterone charms the body into health. It's not a magic potion, although many of my patients claim its effects feel miraculous. Testosterone is just another hormone your aging body finds hard to produce, but this "normal" hormone is packed with a vigorous punch. Your body is worth choosing the right tools to build it to last. With administration of a testosterone prescription designed for your specific needs, along with a diet designed for your bones and a little sweat of the brow, your body could last far into its nineties. The great new is that you *do* have a choice for a healthy and vibrant aging.

What it Really Means to Have a Good Heart

Statistics are grim for men and heart disease. The American Heart Association estimates that ninety thousand men between the ages forty-five and sixty-four die each year from heart attacks or other heart complications. *Ninety thousand* is a tremendous amount of people who more likely than not, could have prevented the onset of heart disease. I believe optimal levels of hormones create a healthy environment for the heart to thrive in. Hormones are the essential building blocks to a healthy and vibrant lifestyle. As I explained in the estrogen chapter, women find themselves facing a shockingly new set of risks as they enter into the years after menopause. Their hormones plummet, and besides feeling crummy, they experience an actual physical crumbling. The same happens with men and low testosterone levels. In the case of testosterone, absence does not make the heart grow fonder. The male heart has a good many cellular receptor sites specifically designed for testosterone. Therefore, it's safe to say that testosterone and the heart are closely related and are a prime example of how one hormone can make or break an organ, in this case, the heart.

Unfortunately, this plain as day fact has been overlooked. For a while, researchers *actually* believed that testosterone was bad medicine for the heart, hence the reason women avoided heart problems up into their sixties while their male counterparts were dropping like flies from heart attacks. Researchers believed estrogen saved the heart while testosterone was a traitor to the same body that produced it. Nothing could be further from the truth. Normal to high levels of testosterone prove to increase a male's life span. As far as the heart is concerned, higher levels of testosterone decrease overall cholesterol levels while maintaining the good cholesterol, HDL, at optimal levels. The measure of HDL is a sure indicator of heart health and with testosterone boosting it to proper levels, the heart is safe from diseases. Beyond this, testosterone has an artery dilating effect, which increases coronary blood flow and permits the heart to receive and release blood easier.

As I said before, testosterone has muscle-enhancing benefits. Our heart is not an exception. The heart works in our waking, physical hours as well as our sleeping hours. It is constantly beating out our life-sustaining blood, and supplying the outer extremities with nourishment and energy. As we grow older, there is a reduction in the rate of blood flow throughout the body, witnessed in the physical evidence of age: graying and loss of hair, skin wrinkling, and nails becoming more brittle. The internal damage is undetectable by the naked eye, although intensely felt by the victim. Blood flow affects so many aspects of every day living. Our memory and sexual arousal depend on blood flow and the nutrients and hormones it carries with it. When restricted, every system suffers, even the tiniest of particles within a cell.

I've had several male patients who complain to me of chest pain. "Roy" said it felt like a vise had a hold of his heart and someone kept cranking the handle. "I think it's killing me." He was right, it was killing him. Roy is one of many who are seized by a distinct pain in the chest, angina, caused by a lack of oxygen to the heart. It's a pain that turns the face ashen white and stricken with fear. It's a reminder that you're one step closer to death. I checked Roy's testosterone levels, which proved what I had already guessed, that they were subnormal, and I prescribed him transdermal testosterone. After three months he came in for a check-up and I asked whether or not the vise was still clamping down on his heart. He smiled and replied, "The only vise I know of is in my garage, on my work bench."

It has been shown that testosterone increases the production of nitric oxide, a natural form of nitroglycerine, the drug taken to alleviate chest pains by opening up the coronary arteries. In a study conducted by Dr. Maurice Lesser, one hundred men who suffered from angina pectoris (spurred by a spasm or blockage of arteries in the heart) were given testosterone injections. Out of the one hundred men, ninety-one showed "moderate to marked" improvement in their chest pain. The frequency and severity of heart attacks diminished greatly. Only *nine* of the one hundred subjects experienced no progress toward a healthier heart and an enhanced quality of life.

Another study indicated that one year of testosterone replacement therapy in hypogonadal and elderly men may have a positive effect on lipid metabolism by lowering overall cholesterol by twenty percent and atherogenic fraction of LDL cholesterol by twenty-five percent. The study showed that the changes in the cholesterol did not negatively affect the level of HDL, which is necessary to maintain a healthy heart.

Many studies, like those above, have witnessed to testosterone's heart healthy effects. It's beyond me that it's not discussed more often as a method of treatment in matters of the heart. Studies dating back to the mid 1970's have shown that men with low levels of testosterone tend to illustrate high cholesterol and triglyceride levels. Since then, study after study has proved that testosterone is designed, in part, to take care of the heart. So where's the hang up? There are plenty of doctors out there, and let me first disclaim, I'm not saying your doctor is not educated, but many doctors are skeptical of hormone replacement therapy. I have found that doctors find themselves in awkward positions when their patients are more aware of current groundbreaking studies than they are. They are at a fork in the road, so to speak, and can either be gracious with the information and make the endeavor to become more knowledgeable for the patient's sake, or they can shun the topic and sway the patient away from sometimes very applicable information. I myself try to take the first approach. I've had many patients who have come to me frustrated that their doctors ignore their requests. What I've noticed is the connotations of the title "doctor" inhibits doctors from admitting they are wrong, and instead they disagree with what they don't understand. We hate the thing that poses a threat to our intelligence.

In truth, testosterone affects the heart in so many different ways. It cleans up the heart's passageways (arteries) by lowering LDL, it causes vasodilatation which allows more blood to the heart, thus lowering the chance of chest pain, and it keeps the HDL at optimal levels. Testosterone and the heart have a long, symbiotic history. If the heart works right, it can pump the bioavailable testosterone to other cellular receptor sites and incite sexual activity or bone health. If testosterone is at optimal levels, then the heart as a whole is a stronger muscle and the rest of our body benefits from its nourishing flow. Yet, even in light of this outstanding proof, many cardiologists still ignore it as possible therapy. Testosterone lowers fibrinogens, serum triglycerides, total cholesterol and LDL cholesterol, and apo A-I lipoprotein, all risk factors of heart disease. Testosterone may be the arrow that hits the bull's eye as far as the heart is concerned, and overlooking its proven benefits is truly a crime against the one thing that manages to keep the body going day after day.

The Smart Hormone

It's funny, who would have thought that testosterone would have been a "smart hormone." Testosterone is sometimes used in the derogatory sense, as if it only controls the muscle bound, oversexed cave man. We hear things like, "He has too much testosterone," or "That's the testosterone speaking." Both comments refer to when a man is overtly sexual or physical. As a society, we feel comfortable reducing the hormones, like estrogen or testosterone, into very shallow and simple definitions. It's not that easy and although testosterone does increase muscle mass and strength and boost a man's sex drive, it also allows men to rationalize and retain information.

Testosterone *is* a smart hormone.

Aging's most obvious and dramatic effects are on the brain. As we get older, a list of factors from diet to medications wear and tear on the brain, resulting in cognitive deterioration, a source for diseases like Alzheimer's. There are two different types of cells in the brain, the neurons and glial cells. We have a finite number of neurons (they don't generally divide and cannot be replaced) and glial cells (which insulate the precious neurons that we have and aid in neuronal transduction). This is why people who have had strokes sometimes never recover, because certain neurons are destroyed.

Neurons operate via chemical messengers called neurotransmitters. In the estrogen chapter I spoke of estrogen's stimulatory effect on probably the most important of the neurotransmitters, acetylcholine, but there are others, which include dopamine, norepinephrine, serotonin, epinephrine, and histamine. These neurotransmitters, like neurons, diminish over time. The bridges or synapses that link and process messages between a neuron and a neurotransmitter also decline with age. With the depreciation of the messengers and the messages, the end result is a slower wit, longer reaction time, and the inability to recall names and places.

I think the saddest portrait of age is of a person locked away from his or her own mind and memories. We spend years experiencing life, but for all those good and bad experiences, they have no merit if they cannot be found in the jumbled mess of declining neurons, neurotransmitters, and synapses.

With more and more people living well into their eighties, medicine has to be on its toes to meet their cognitive needs. It's estimated that Alzheimer's disease claims over four million people in the United States alone and is the most common cause of dementia. Alzheimer's is recognized by abnormal clumps, referred to as senile plaques and irregular knots, called neurofibrillary tangles, of brain cells. The plaque is usually formed by longer forms of a beta-amyloid peptide, referred to as beta-amyloid-42. These two aspects of Alzheimer's jumble the memory and the learning processes. A healthy brain has a sense of order about it, like a fine-tuned racecar engine. In contrast, a brain affected by Alzheimer's looks like a tortured mess of tendrils.

Researchers are finding increasingly more information that may provide salvation for the mind. Sex steroids have been the subject of memory research for a decade or so and estrogen has proved to be a veritable ally to the brain, but what about testosterone? Many scientists and doctors have asked the same question. There are receptors in the brain specially designed for testosterone and it would seem these receptors indicate that testosterone has some sort of cerebral purpose. Studies have confirmed this. In the Department of Neurology at Oregon Health Sciences University in Portland, Oregon, a group of researchers studied the relationship between working memory and sex steroid concentrations and whether or not sex steroid supplementation would alter age-related loss of working memory. To compare the results of the study before and after, the men and women subjects were given a Subject Ordered Pointing Test (SOP) before being given hormone supplementation; in which case, the older proved to do much worse than the younger subjects. What was fascinating about the result of the study after hormone supplementation is that testosterone enhanced the working memory in men while estrogen seemed to provide no improvement in women. In the men, testosterone and estrogen effects were correlative, although working memory faired better in a higher testosterone-to-estrogen ratio. Testosterone had the power to accentuate working memory, and it seems possible that beyond just working memory, testosterone may enhance other important aspects of cognition.

A ground-breaking study has revealed that testosterone may be a protective accessory to the brain in evading Alzheimer's disease. Above, I described how Alzheimer's destroys any rhyme or reason a healthy mind once possessed. The media has referred to it as the disease of the century and although we have found methods to alleviate, somewhat, it's vandalism in the brain, we still haven't discovered the actual reason why it happens and thus, we have discovered no cure. Researchers are furiously trying to find ways to prevent it from happening and it seems hormones may be the key that unlocks the door on the mysteries of this debilitating illness. At the Rockefeller University and the Well Medical College of Cornell University, researchers have found that extra testosterone added to nerve cells inhibited the growth of plaque formation in the brain. This senile plaque formation is the hallmark indication of Alzheimer's disease. In rat and mice neurons, testosterone treatment decreased the secretion of beta-amyloid peptides (the proteins responsible for the harmful plaque formation) by 30 to 45 percent, while increasing the secretion of harmless fragments. They compared these findings to treatment with other kinds of steroidal hormones, cholesterol and corticosterone, which offered no reduction in beta-amyloid levels, thereby confirming the hypothesis that beta-amyloid-precursor-protein metabolism may be sensitive specifically to the actions of the sex steroid, testosterone.

Month after month, new research pops up and offers the latest word on Alzheimer's disease. Lately, that word seems to be testosterone. The above studies along with others raise the possibility that Alzheimer's can be stifled at its onset and that hormones play a vital role in preventing it. Alzheimer's is an illness that is rarely seen in those under 50. It is no coincidence that it correlates with the depression of the hormones that sustain us in our youth. These "normal" diseases that we evaded while we were in our youth, we seem to attract as we push into our sixties. I want you to know, there is nothing "normal" about being sick or feeling not up to learning a new trick. I hear over and over again a general apathy toward aging and disease as if it's not a question of choice but rather a "have to" situation. I'm writing this book to dispel the myth about "obligatory aging." I'm not about to give up the ghost and neither should you. New research qualifies you to live longer, and hormone supplementation happens to be a large bulk of that research. Longevity is not wishful thinking. Your mind is a powerful and essential part of your being. It mandates how your organs and emotions react to both positive and negative stimuli. The years ahead of you are worth remembering, and testosterone may be the essential tool to keep your brain running like a fine-tuned engine rather than a muddled mess. Take the initiative to live longer. Reading this book is the first step, now the ball is in your court. For the sake of your body and mind, don't drop the ball.

Getting the Prostate Under Control

Testosterone in association with the prostate has been subject of much research as well as much controversy. A couple of decades ago, the word prostate had a foreign ring to it. Now it's a household name, as common to men as the words Monday Night Football. So, why the sudden interest? As I've mentioned before, we're living longer. As the years build upon one another, they topple down on our healthy organs or glands. In the case of the prostate, a tremendous number of cases ranging in severity have popped up over the last several decades. Prostate cancer, unlike many cancers, is somewhat stealthy in its telltale signs. Interestingly, some men never know they have cancer and only after dying of other causes, their autopsies reveal cancerous growths on the prostate. However, if the prostatic cancer is found soon enough, it can be effectively treated. All in all, the likelihood of a man having problems with his prostate is quite high. But, before I get into the fallacies of the prostate, I think it is important to understand its geography and purpose.

The prostate is a chestnut shaped gland tucked behind the pubic bone, in front of the rectum, below the bladder. It ranges about three centimeters in width and weighs about twenty grams. The seminal vesicles, attached to the prostate, produce components that, when mixed with the prostate fluid, generates semen. Tubes from the testicles carry sperm to the prostate where it is all mixed together. The fluid, added to the sperm, gives it more agility and mobility. Not only this, but this potassium/enzyme-rich fluid also nourishes and harbors the sperm while it waits for release.

The prostate also wraps around the urethra, the tube that carries urine from the bladder to the penis. This major thoroughfare travels right through the center of the prostate, and it is this relationship that causes the major prostatic problems men experience as they get older.

Before I explain the maladies of the prostate, I want to stress now as well as later that optimal levels of testosterone are the prostate's best resource to a healthy longevity. It's only when testosterone levels decline that the prostate suffers from the alterations I'll describe below. Prostate cancer or an enlarged prostate is an age-related disease. When boys experience testosterone peaks, and when testosterone is at its highest, prostates are also healthy. It is only when age begins to rob the body of testosterone that complications with the prostate arise.

As I mentioned before, the risk of prostate cancer increases in every man as he puts on the years. But the most common prostate disorder is benign prostatic hyperplasia (BPH), a noncancerous condition that may cause substantial growth and discomfort. The prostate has a normal growth spurt during puberty when it increases in weight and doubles in size. During a man's forties or fifties, there is a good chance that his prostate will experience another spurt in growth, although this time it's considered abnormal. The American Foundation for Urologic Disease estimates that 50 percent of all men, fifty or above, face the complications of BPH; the percentage increases to 80 percent once they hit the age of eighty. The prostate can enlarge from 20 grams up to 150 grams, and this enlargement puts stress on the urethra and in worst case scenarios can cause total blockage of urine. Although BPH is nonmalignant, it's quite common and the more minor symptoms feel anything but benign. When the prostate enlarges, it can cause one or more uncomfortable consequences. The list is long and unattractive:

> Frequent need to urinate.
> Nocturnal urinating.
> Difficulty urinating.
> Urgency to urinate accompanied by difficulty to empty bladder.
> Weaker stream of urine.
> Even after emptying bladder, still feeling bladder fullness.
> Incontinence.

Doesn't sound too appealing, does it? The sad truth is, whether we like it or not, the odds are that many men will one day experience two to three of the above symptoms.

There are several different treatment options for BPH. Medications, like Proscar, can either shrink or relax the prostate tissue, alleviating the pressure on the urethra. Herbal supplements like Saw Palmetto or Pygeum have also been shown to positively affect the symptoms of BPH. Ten percent of men in the United States will have prostate surgery at one point their life. The standard procedure is called transurethral resection of the prostate (TURP). The surgeon uses an endoscope, a tube with a camera and sharp instrument attached to it, to cut away excess prostate tissue.

Although BPH is the most common foe to the prostate, prostate cancer is also a veritable enemy. Unlike other cancers, which spread like wildfire, this type of cancer is very sluggish in its development and can actually take more than a decade to meander out of the prostate and become dangerous. Of course, no man wants to wait until that happens, and would rather trap the cancer before it traps him.

A mandatory, yearly breast exam for women over the age of thirty-five is a given; I advise my male patients who are forty-five years of age or older to also get a yearly prostate exam. When the prostate becomes aggravated it produces large amounts of a protein called prostate specific antigen (PSA). Although this test is relatively accurate, I always suggest, just in case my patient is one of those rare cases that the PSA is not triggered by the cancer, that he have a Digital Rectal Exam (DRE). This procedure entails a physician manually feeling the prostate gland for lumps or hardened cancerous growths.

With the American Cancer Association estimating that 200,000 patients each year will be diagnosed with prostate cancer and that 41,000 will actually die, there is a desperate need to find ways to halt or cure the cancer. There are different ways to manage prostate cancer, the most severe being radical prostatectomy. In fifty percent of patients, this removal of the prostate causes lifelong impotence or incontinence. Other non-invasive, less consequential ways of handling prostate cancer are found in herbal supplementation. The newest researched over-the-counter herbal supplement, PC-SPES (PC short for prostate cancer and spes is the Latin word for hope) has shown promising results for prostate cancer. It significantly lowers prostate specific antigen levels, and in some exceptional cases has sent the cancer into remission. In a 1999 study published in the International Journal of Oncology, researchers followed sixteen patients with advanced prostate cancer, taking 2.7 grams of PC-SPES. At the three-month check-up, ten of the sixteen patients showed a more than 50 percent decline in their PSA levels. There is hope in PC-SPES although we still have questions regarding who it is best for and what its long-term results are.

Now that you have a fair idea of the prostate and its purpose and detriments, I want to discuss the testosterone predicament.

Androgens have been thought to play a role in the origination and development of prostate disease. I believe this to be far from the truth. Androgens do not cause prostate cancer. They may cause cell proliferation once the cancer is already there, but there is no definitive proof, *anywhere*, that androgens, specifically testosterone and its stronger offspring, DHT, initiate cancer in the prostate. A DHT patch is actually in the process of being approved by the FDA. If it was so dangerous to the prostate, I doubt it would even be up for consideration. If testosterone was so dangerous to the prostate gland, then it seems that most young men who have higher testosterone concentrations in the blood would be suffering prostate problems and have higher PSA levels. This is not the case. Studies have shown that BPH and prostate cancer do not correlate to high testosterone levels and neither do PSA levels. BPH and prostate cancer are diseases that age instigates, and since we already know testosterone declines as men get older, it seems to have a valid alibi.

On the other hand, estradiol leaps into action as men age, and studies have shown estradiol is the more likely culprit. Nothing is set in stone of course, studies and hypotheses are still going on and being made, but a fair body of evidence is pointing in that direction. Some studies have shown that estrogen levels are higher in men with enlarged prostates (BPH) while the men with the least amount of enlargement have higher testosterone levels. If the levels of estrogen are high and the testosterone levels low, the risk of developing BPH increases significantly. This may seem to have nothing to do with prostate cancer, but I believe if estrogen is able to pester the prostate in this manner, it seems viable that is can be a factor in the development of prostate cancer.

There are studies that indicate high levels of estrogen and low levels of testosterone are indicative of prostate cancer. Just this year, the journal *Prostate* reported that patients with a high Gleason score for prostate cancer had low testosterone levels. Another study in the journal, *Drugs and Aging*, two researchers from the Department of Medical Oncology at the St. Bartholomew's and the Royal London Hospital School of Medicine, West Smithfield, England, evaluated 34 studies of prostate cancer in relation to testosterone and came to the conclusion that there was really no convincing evidence that testosterone instigated prostate complications and cancer. Rather, they believe that if there is any correlation between the two of them, it's an indirect link of lifestyle. In all actuality, prostate cancers arising in men with low serum testosterone levels are more malignant and frequently unresponsive to hormones.

Once cancer is found, doctors must determine whether it has spread or not and therefore how to treat it. If it has remained in the prostate, then doctors may opt to remove the prostate or treat it with radiation. If it has spread outside of the prostate, doctors usually induce a hormonal therapy that does the opposite of what this entire book is about; it suppresses testosterone and DHT, testosterone's potent derivative. This technique is called androgen blockade. Deprived of testosterone, the prostate atrophies, giving the cancer a less stable environment to survive in. It therefore seems to halt the cancerous growth, albeit, for only a year or two. Since some cells are independent of testosterone, they survive beyond the hormonal blockade; thus the cancer returns.

We should be aware of BPH and prostate cancer, but not wary of testosterone therapy. There is a reason men have evaded prostate cancer up until their forties or fifties and I believe it is because testosterone levels are where they should be. Optimal testosterone levels are perhaps the best omens for prostatic health. When they decline, anything is fair game, and the prostate seems to be no exception.

Fine Tune Yourself for the Years to Come

> *It has saved my marriage. Before, I thought I was going mad. It seemed my world was crumbling beneath my feet. I felt exposed and angry at my vulnerability…I felt dangerous to myself and to others. I was utterly alone.*
> —Reed, 54

Remember the story I began this chapter with, of the man who had it all? I want to finish that story now.

One of his friends watched patiently as this man presented more and more symptoms that were all too familiar and finally decided to intervene. He recommended that he visit me. The man found it so exasperating that his lack of restraint was obvious, he refused for months. In the meantime, his marriage fell into disrepair and his waist grew in size several inches. He tried to double his work out time but he found that he grew more and more tired with each passing month. He knew these were the residual signs of aging but found no relief in knowing this was a common occurrence. He was at an impasse—he felt he was on a one way street to a dead end.

When he finally visited me, he grudgingly listened, arms folded, facial expression stony, as I explained, step by step, what was happening to him. I recounted his downward spiral, verbatim, without his having to tell me anything. I postulated that he felt anxious and depressed, that his pants felt a little tighter at the waist, that he felt sluggish and listless, like the world kept on moving at its same pace while he kept moving slower and slower. When I was done, his expression and manner had lost its determined disinterest. He had a look of incredulity at my ability to read him like a book. I assured him that I was no psychic but that he was not alone, in fact he was one of many who visit me weekly with the same dilemmas. I asked him, if he could take something natural that would boost his lean muscle mass while reducing his fat, that within months would dissipate the depression and frustration that had become second nature to him, which would greaten his interest in sex and assist in the performance, would he take it? What if he could take something that did all the formerly mentioned things, in addition to boosting heart health, bone density, and his overall energy level, would he do it? His answer was an emphatic yes. We tested his free testosterone and estradiol levels and determined to put him on testosterone, along with Arimidex to quell the surge of estrogen that seemed to prevent the testosterone he had from working properly.

Months after our first visit, I found a renewed man sitting in front of me. He said business was great, as usual, and he and his wife were going on a second honeymoon. He said the testosterone was a godsend, like some miraculous manna. I laughed, because this manna happened to be something he had since his fetal stage. We take for granted our endocrine system until our hormones sink below their normal levels. It becomes very obvious when all the health benefits they once offered fade and are replaced with the uncomfortable side effects of aging. I suppose the effect of supplemented testosterone, to a deprived man, feels miraculous, as if his starved receptors received a sudden jolt of vitality. I believe men, like women, should not go without the essential hormones that once added spice to their life during their twenties and thirties. Testosterone is as essential as air itself, and I'm afraid to say, men have been kept in the dark far too long about its decline and their own age-related andropause. Testosterone has been a taboo subject, something that controversy has gravitated to throughout the years. It has been wrongly accused as the guilty party behind prostate cancer and as an abused substance of body builders. Women have been told it will cause unwanted hair growth, no matter what the dosage. And at one time, doctors and researchers actually believed it was dangerous to the male body, thus men suffered more heart attacks than women. It remains clear to me and my patients, both male and female, that testosterone, throughout all the false accusations, is a boon to the body. It protects the body against heart disease, osteoporosis, and prostate cancer. It also revitalizes muscles and skin and it significantly enhances the quality of life. In effect, testosterone can literally transform an ailing man into his healthy mirror image. Age may flip the hormone switch to a lower setting, but now you have the education of the resources to flip the switch back to where it was in your more youthful, energetic years.

Testosterone:
The Female's side of the Story

Testosterone completely shot my libido up. It seemed I wanted sex all the time.
—Felicia, 43

I heard that testosterone caused abnormal hair growth. When my doctor prescribed it, all I could imagine is what I would look like with a beard in a new job as a side-show act. Boy, was I wrong. I feel like a butterfly hatched from a long cocooned sleep. I feel sexy and colorful—a far cry from the circus act I imagined.
—Kharen, 56

It's somewhat humorous that there are women out there who blame the world's ills on testosterone without the knowledge that this same "chauvinist" hormone actually resides in their body and provides some very helpful and enjoyable aspects, like bone health and sex drive, to name just a few. And just as men are shocked by the idea that their bodies thrive with help from estrogen, women, too, are a bit stunned by the news that, whether they like it or not and even in this day and age, they can't quite make it without testosterone. Testosterone levels in the female body are about 10 percent of the amount in men, but that 10 percent makes all the difference. It has been found to enhance sex drive and mood, while working to maintain bone health and lean muscle mass. Testosterone is as essential to female health and well-being as are progesterone and estrogen, yet for some reason, it is a far less prescribed hormone. Unfortunately, testosterone has been intentionally left off the female hormone roster, and this exclusion leaves a woman not quite altogether herself. There seems to be an irrational fear that pervades our society pertaining to women and supplemental testosterone. Some people are sure that women administered testosterone will undergo a masculine transformation. Hair will grow on the face, the voice will deepen, and even the personality will take on a more masculine temperament. I'm here to tell you this is silly paranoia brought on by the lack of research and an overactive imagination. Nevertheless, you wouldn't believe the aversion displayed by some of my female patients when I prescribe them what has been falsely proclaimed as the "male" hormone. Once they have been on testosterone for a few months, they're singing quite a different tune.

All the above adverse side effects only occur at high, irresponsible dosages. A capable doctor will tailor a hormone program around the specific needs of each patient. I use levels from blood tests as well as a woman's description of symptoms to calculate what dosages will effectively and safely urge her levels up into more youthful ranges. After about six weeks, the patient has a follow-up appointment where I check her levels and assess whether I need to adjust her dosages or not. Studies that convey concern about women taking testosterone or that have shown ill-effects, used too high of dosages. Tragically, these studies received a large amount of press, while other studies, dating way back to the late 1950's that claimed testosterone enhanced sexuality and energy, were buried and forgotten.

Sadly, it's not just the layman that incorrectly considers testosterone replacement in women as something not only unneeded, but even dangerous. There are also doctors who have perpetuated this myth. This is why only a very small percentage of women are actually getting the full and complete benefit from their hormone regimen. Without testosterone, I feel women are perhaps getting the main course but are missing the spice that makes it interesting and palatable. I'm writing this chapter separate from the main testosterone chapter because I feel women suffer their own testosterone deficiency. On top of menopause, they suffer a form of andropause, and although women receive prescriptions of estrogen and progesterone, they have to battle social protocols and unfounded fears to be supplemented with testosterone. Here I stress, testosterone *must* be replaced just as estrogen and progesterone are. This chapter is to encourage women to rise above rumors instigated more by inertia than ignorance (doctors sometimes get in a habit of sticking with the old rather than exploring the new), and enjoy the full spectrum of hormone replacement therapy.

In the Mood?

Testosterone is formed in both the ovaries and the adrenal glands. It travels through the body via the blood, but most is attached to the protein, sex hormone-binding globulin. Basically, only one to three percent of testosterone is free to link up with tissues and produce the hormonal response desired. Even in that small amount, there is a time-related drop in testosterone that begins after a woman's 20's, but this decrease is augmented when a woman passes through menopause and her ovaries become dormant along with a slowing down of her adrenal glands. Testosterone production slackens as well as the adrenal glands' manufacturing of DHEA and androstenedione (steroids that convert into testosterone). When these declines take place, a woman feels a stark absence in the feelings of sexual arousal. Basically, testosterone is the stuff desire is made of. Just as testosterone flips a switch in boys during puberty, testosterone also aids girls in their sexual awakening. It is testosterone that stimulates the growth of pubic and underarm hair. It has specific receptors located in the breasts, vagina, and clitoris. Testosterone's presence stimulates the sensations that women feel in sexual situations. It's basically the tool that turns a woman on.

When testosterone levels drop and sexual desire dissipates, women find they are trapped in a medical world unwilling to help. Women find they are up against conventional wisdom that states their lack of sexual desire is due to a mental block, rather than a block in their testosterone production. I have encountered many a female patient frustrated and humiliated by the care they have received from their general practitioner or gynecologist. These patients don't understand how this "neurosis" developed only after they started the perimenopause, menopause, and postmenopausal process. Dr. Susan Rako, in her book <u>The Hormone of Desire: The Truth About Sexuality, Menopause and Testosterone</u>, couldn't have said it better: "Menopause is a journey through poorly charted waters and most physicians approach the possibility of prescribing supplementary testosterone for women suffering symptoms of its deficiency with the resistance and ignorance of sailors who believed the earth was flat, and that if they proceeded to sail on, they would fall off."

This chapter is specifically for you women butting your heads against traditional medicine. Your sudden sexual dysfunction is not a mental problem, nor does it lie in uncharted waters. There is research that confirms testosterone supplementation helps sexual apathy as well as aiding in a number of other facets that influence sexual appetite, like mood and energy. I want to supply you women with enough clinical ammunition so that, when a doctor tells you there is no relation between your lack of sexual longing and low testosterone levels, you can pull out this book and point to the sources that say differently.

In women, testosterone levels actually fall over time. Levels peak while women are in their 20's and slowly slide into lower levels with each passing year. Once they hit menopause, testosterone could be at an all time low and is only magnified by symptoms of estrogen and progesterone deficiencies. The most prominent effect of testosterone depletion is the slackening of sexual appetite. One of my female patients described this as a deadening. "I just feel like that part of my life is over. I've tried everything from the Kama Sutra to just plain smut and nothing seems to awaken my comatose sexual desire." After a few months on testosterone, during her follow-up, she smiled slyly when I asked her about her sex life "Let's just say a miracle has occurred, it's been resurrected."

Women experience a gradual sexual decline as they grow older. Later this is coupled with the onset of menopause, when women experience an even higher rate of coital infrequency. Estrogen replacement can help only to the degree that it decreases bothersome menopausal symptoms and increases vaginal moistness. The libido, however, is primarily the responsibility of testosterone. Study after study affirms that midlife sexual dysfunction is easily abated with testosterone administration. With testosterone supplementation, women experience not only a sexual surge, but it seems to put their sex life into full throttle (it's not unusual for women to experience a resurgence of visual fantasies and multiple orgasms when taking some form of testosterone). Many studies have compared sexual parameters as they relate to estrogen therapy alone or estrogen replacement coupled with testosterone therapy. All studies seem to agree that estrogen alone has no influence on a woman's sexual health, but when combined with testosterone, it's amazing the change women experience in their attitude and ability. The two hormones work in tandem to create a healthy physical and emotional environment. In a 1998 double-blind, randomized study, twenty postmenopausal women were given either estrogen or an estrogen/androgen combination. After four to eight weeks, women on the estrogen/androgen combination had a marked increase in sexual sensation and desire compared to the women on estrogen alone. Another point of interest from this particular study is that the estrogen-only treatment seemed to directly correlate with an increase in sex hormone-binding globulin (the protein that binds to testosterone, immobilizing it and making it worthless). The opposite was found in the estrogen/androgen study. Here SHBG actually decreased, freeing up testosterone, which resulted in a higher rate of sexual interest and activity.

This study is particularly interesting because of the implications that estrogen replacement may be somewhat of an inhibitor to the remaining testosterone a woman creates after menopause. I'm not indicating that women go off estrogen because it boosts the production of SHBG, there are too many valuable resources estrogen provides to the heart, bone, and vagina. What I do suggest is that women take testosterone along with their other hormones. As we saw in the study above, testosterone curbs estrogen's influence on the overproduction of SHBG. This way, the testosterone you supplement your body with is more able to remain free and active for bodily tissues, while estrogen is also able to aid the bone, heart, and mind.

While many women are solely on estrogen replacement, there are some that receive the added benefits of natural progesterone; but only a handful receives the advantages of testosterone. There are so many women led to believe that their sexual listlessness resides in their head, a purely psychological setback, and therefore are treated accordingly. For many of these women, this kind of therapy is frustrating and embarrassing. A good indicator for testosterone deficiency is a loss of sexual responsiveness in all phases: not only sexual arousal from a partner, but also from self. I had a patient—we'll call her "Linda"—who felt guilty over her passionate dismay at her husband's advances. She hadn't always felt that way, but this new negativity toward intimacy seemed to create a rift in their marriage. She went to counseling for several months, and later described it to me as "therapy that was like hitting her head against the wall"—it offered no clue to her sexual inhibition. I measured her total and free testosterone levels and discovered they were quite low. After the proper dosage and several months later, Linda called to say she was no longer banging her head against the wall and her husband thanks me for it.

Other great side effects of testosterone replacement that accentuate sexuality are energy and optimism. I believe that vitality and enhanced mood alone can boost a woman's sex drive. A woman has a challenging time feeling desire when she is overwhelmed by fatigue and depression. I think the elevation in these two factors help aid in sexual contentedness. Several tests have indicated that testosterone bolsters optimism and vigor in surgically menopausal women. In a 1988 study, researchers found that intramuscular administration of testosterone added to estrogen replacement resulted in test subjects feeling more able to cope with daily stresses. They also felt a larger rush of energy and optimism than the women solely supplemented with estrogen. Thirteen years later, another study, published in the *New England Journal of Medicine*, related the results of transdermal administration in oophorectomized (removal of one or both ovaries) women. The randomized clinical study was done on seventy-five women aged 31-56 who had undergone a hysterectomy and bilateral salpingo-oophorectomy one to ten years previous and who had serum total and free testosterone levels below normal. After a four-week baseline period, the women were placed on three, consecutive twelve-week supplement regimens: either placebo, 150 mcg of testosterone, or 300 mcg of testosterone. Mood was assessed by the "Psychological General Well Being Index," a questionnaire designed to gauge vitality, self-control, well-being, general health, depressed mood, and anxiety. Women on the highest amount of testosterone scored the highest on the questionnaire as far as improvement in mood and depression.

Testosterone is a potent remedy for sexual dysfunction. This segment is for all women whose sexual comfort has been neglected and overlooked. It's time to ask your doctor to measure your testosterone levels. If he or she is opposed, find someone who will. With prudent judgment and monitoring, you can again feel sexy and content in your sensuality. Age does not mean abstinence and it certainly does not mean displeasure. I believe intimacy is as necessary to health as is the right diet and enough sleep. If you are one of the many women out there experiencing a sexual slump, snap out of it, and have your testosterone levels checked. You could experience a miracle also, and witness your own sexual reawakening.

At the Mercy of Hormones?

Most people have been taught to consume calcium by drinking so many glasses of milk each day. Most people know that vitamin D somehow affects the bone. But what a lot people don't know is that our sex hormones play a substantial role in the delicate balance of bone reproduction. You can drink glass after glass of milk each day and pop vitamin D all you want, but as we get older, our hormones will decline and our bones, in consequence, will become weaker.

How many times have you seen an older person warped by age. It's a sobering portrait of a body without the proper defenses to ward off what aging can do to the bones. Doctors and researchers have observed how our bones survive over the years by a battery of reconstruction. Our bones are dynamic works of art that need maintenance and understanding to maintain a proper equilibrium. As I have explained in previous chapters, we have a construction crew of specialized cells called osteoblasts and osteoclasts that work in conjunction with one another to either build or tear down bone. When our hormones decline, which they most certainly do, the equilibrium between these cells breaks down, and osteoclasts run amuck, reabsorping more bone than what is being made. There is no coincidence between bone loss and gaining years. There is also no twist of fate that when hormones are added back to the female body, there is a remarkable increase in bone density. I showed you evidence of this in the estrogen and progesterone chapters.

Collecting research now shows that when testosterone is added to a woman's hormonal treatment, bone density improves more dramatically than if she were left on estrogen or progesterone supplementation alone. Doctors are finding that levels of bioavailable testosterone are predictors, in men *and* women, of height loss and subsequent vertebral fractures. Other studies have shown that small amounts of testosterone added to estrogen increased bone formation by 50 percent over a three-month period. By including just a small amount of testosterone to your hormone replacement program, you could potentially boost your bone-loss prevention efforts by a good 41 percent. Those percentages alone should be enough to make you call your doctor for a lab appointment.

The estrogen/androgen combination has proved over and over to be a formidable enemy to osteoporosis. One of the best examples of its awesome capabilities to combat bone loss while fostering new bone is a study done by Davis and his colleagues in 1995. Over a two-year, single-blind trial of thirty-four menopausal women, these researchers observed the bone mineral density in juxtaposition with either estradiol replacement therapy or estradiol/testosterone replacement therapy. The pellets were inserted every three months and at the end of the study, bone mineral density was measured by using dual-energy x-ray absorptiometry. Both hormone treatments increased total body-, lumbar vertebrae-, and hip bone mineral density compared to when the women first began the programs, but the real clincher was the results for the estrogen/androgen combination therapy. In the women on this program there was a trend of faster growth with a more significant increase in total body-, vertebral-, and trochanteric mineral density than the women on estradiol alone. The androgen made all the difference without canceling out any of estrogen's stimulatory factors.

The recipe for bone health has been missing an ingredient in most HRT programs. Testosterone has been overlooked or pushed aside as something unessential to the female body (which I find amusing, since she's been manufacturing it on her own for so many years, and the body never does anything without motivation or purpose).

Testosterone is a bonus for bone health, but too many women never get that extra boost. I'm surprised over and over when women come to my office on synthetic hormones, and have never heard of natural hormones, let alone testosterone. Their vitality has plunged and their sex life is null, but what they *don't* know is worse—their bones are wasting away. You do have the right to request, first of all, natural hormones, and second, all the essential hormones.

More Side Benefits of Testosterone For Women

Many times when people discuss hormone replacement therapy they stress the side effects, yet when a woman's testosterone is restored to optimal and prime levels women experience what I like to call "side benefits." Some of these pleasant side benefits include the revitalization of skin texture. Testosterone increases the collagen content and elasticity to prevent wrinkles. Other aesthetic improvements reside in women attaining that youthful shape they once had. Testosterone adds muscle back to support the curves you once took pride in. Your fat to muscle ratio flips, and you'll notice a more toned and defined figure. Not only that, you'll discover you have more energy and desire to workout and be active. Your strength and endurance will surprise you. You won't fatigue as easily and your joints won't ache like they used to.

Studies have shown that testosterone may also have cardiovascular protective functions. A combination of testosterone and estrogen has been shown to have beneficial effects of the cardiovascular system, especially concerning lipids, atherogenesis, and vasodilation. It has been shown to improve vasomotor stability and lower triglyceride levels. Testosterone, like progesterone, is absolutely necessary to add to your estrogen replacement regimen. When all three are combined, a woman can feel herself again. She'll experience a reawakening, not only in her spirits, but also in her skin and the shape of her body. We usually refer to young women as being in full bloom, yet I've seen many a woman under the influence of a complete hormone treatment with testosterone, estrogen, and progesterone as the headlining hormones—literally bloom like that of a perennial blossom.

I urge you to discover the nourishing qualities that these essential hormones have on the outside and inside of your body. They are the fuel on which your vital organs and tissues thrive. I believe hormones are truly the stuff that allows you to grow young and healthy with the years.

Testosterone: The Female Hormone

Testosterone, almost always referred to as the "male hormone," is a misnomer. Testosterone is as much a female hormone, and if anyone tells you differently, they haven't studied their general human biology. Society as a whole feels safer when things are in compartments: estrogen is a female hormone; testosterone is a male hormone, thus the uproar and obstinacy over testosterone supplementation in women. It's time to break free of the constriction in simple thinking. The human body is more complex than clear-cut definitions. Testosterone happens to be both a female and male hormone. If a woman is suffering from malnutrition, we feed her. If a woman is naked, we clothe her. If a woman is testosterone deficient, the popular response has been to ignore her, but no longer. Your health deserves first-rate care, and your sexuality specifically needs attention. We've seen the token portraits of a "dried-up" middle-aged woman who has become stingy with her sexuality. It is not stinginess, only an easily remedied testosterone deficiency. You're not washed up, or done in. You have years ahead of you that just need to be spiced up with the right ingredient. You have the curiosity, that's why you're reading this book—now you need a nudge. Well, here it is:

Testosterone was like fertilizer—in the years that I've been taking it, I feel taller and brighter and fresher than I have in a long time.
—Judy age 55

I never thought I would say this again…but I love sex!
—Mary age 59

…and the energy, I actually thought my doctor laced my cream with some sort of illegal stimulant. I never thought I would feel this good.
—Isabel age 61

Thyroid:
Rethinking the Thyroid

I remember a time when I felt absolutely lifeless. I felt drained of energy and drive. I gained fifteen pounds. I went to several doctors, who either prescribed me some form of antidepressant or brushed me off as being a hypochondriac. I felt worse on the antidepressants and I was frustrated with the lack of help or sympathy I was receiving from my health care.
—Lisa, 39

I have encountered so many people who can honestly say, in lieu of seeing almost every kind of doctor there is out there, from endocrinologist to aromatherapist, they are truly unhealthy and unhappy. They have complaint after complaint, and although their hormone levels seem just about right and their doctors can't pinpoint exactly what it is that ails them, they are positive they are not in good health. But they are, for the most part, except for one small, but significant, adjustment, their thyroids.

A description like the one above is not far from what many people in the United States, especially women, feel these days. When Lisa was referred to me, she viewed me with a skepticism she had developed from her previous health care experiences. Her story was not unusual to me and she seemed baffled at my curiosity and probing questions. I measured her TSH (thyroid-stimulating hormone) level, along with her free T3 and T4 levels. She was definitely suffering from an insufficiency in thyroid, although this was the first time anyone had mentioned her thyroid. Many doctors measured her TSH levels (I'll explain what that is later), along with other standard tests, and found that her levels were "normal." In spite of her normal levels, I treated her anyway with a natural thyroid hormone. She was used to it being something "in her mind," and was relieved to find out that it was her free T-3 levels that were out of whack and not her head. After three weeks, she felt better. "I can actually wake up in the morning and look forward to seeing my husband and going to work." After two months, her added pounds began to fall off. At her follow-up appointment she had lost ten of the fifteen pounds she had gained, the dark circles under eyes had disappeared, and she smiled. "I'm going shopping after our visit to celebrate how good I look and feel." It's important to understand that many doctors will treat blood levels rather than symptoms. I suppose it feels safer to them, but in the mean time, healthcare—I mean true healthcare, caring for the person, not the lab test, is going downhill.

Lisa suffered from one of the most misdiagnosed illnesses patients and doctors are faced with daily. I believe that the thyroid may be one of the most misunderstood and probably one of the most overlooked hormones in the entire endocrine system. More often than not, patients are misread or perhaps their symptoms are merely overlooked, allowing their hypothyroidism (underactive thyroid) to go unchecked or unaltered. Unfortunately, hypothyroidism unchecked can only worsen.

In Dr. Gerald S. Levey's article "Hypothyroidism: A Treacherous Masquerader," he refers to the illness as a subtle disease that alludes doctors. It is basically the melting pot of symptoms. Often, thyroid insufficiency or hypothyroidism is misconstrued in people over fifty or sixty as normal symptoms of aging. Fatigue, slower speech, forgetfulness, weight gain, depression, and the tendency to feel cold are all facets normally, yet erroneously, associated with aging. The orthodox medical community will usually try to treat these symptoms in younger patients, but feel it unnecessary to do the same for their older patients. If you are a person who has reached that age when time seems to have crept up on you and you recognize the above symptoms, yet have been greeted with the same reserved, "fact-of-life" medical resignation that Lisa had received, then this chapter is for you.

You do not have to grow old needlessly.

A woman is more likely to experience hypothyroid symptoms, with the incidence increasing, as she gets older. The problem here is that many times symptoms of hypothyroidism overlap with those of perimenopause and menopause. Although a woman may be supplemented with estrogen and progesterone to eliminate her menopausal symptoms, some complications may seem invariable and stubborn even with their addition. I remember a patient, a teacher, whose estrogen and progesterone levels were restored to normal, yet she couldn't shake her depression and fatigue. "I couldn't focus on my lessons. I had a hard time being creative with my students and because I lacked attention span, I couldn't really capture the interest of my students. All I wanted to do is stay in bed. I had no idea how significant the thyroid was until I started taking it. What a relief to find a doctor not stuck in the Middle Ages." It took her several doctors and several medicinal regimens to finally get referred to me. Her symptoms were so classic—hair falling out, brittle fingernails, coarse skin, and lethargy—I was surprised no one had thought to check her thyroid. When a woman suffers from hypothyroidism, the menopausal process becomes a whole other animal. And since the symptoms are similar (i.e. forgetfulness, depression, mood swings, muscle weakness, change in skin or hair texture, sleep disturbances, anxiety or irritability, palpitations, and irregular periods), many doctors overlook the thyroid and prescribe the normal menopause symptom-curing hormones. As I discussed in previous chapters, estrogen and progesterone are necessary for heart health and osteoporosis deterrence and for many women, they do the trick in eliminating the bothersome menopausal symptoms; but for those women who cannot shake depression and fatigue even after supplementation of estrogen and progesterone, their doctors should take the initiative and check their thyroid levels. I believe more often than not, they will find their levels are "low-normal" or insufficient. If they are low-normal, the doctor will brush over them without notice since they still fall in the "normal" range. Throughout this chapter and the rest of the book you will find the recurrent theme of restoring levels to *optimal* ranges.

Like all our essential hormones, our thyroid levels decrease as we age. Thyroid insufficiency or hypothyroidism is a quite common occurrence: one out of ten women and one out of twenty men suffer from its complications. It's actually more common than you would think, but the problem is that it usually goes undetected. Studies have shown that even when the blood tests say otherwise, a good part, possibly surpassing one-forth, of America is hypothyroid or thyroid insufficient. One study in particular, reported in the *Journal of the American Geriatric Society*, attested to the above findings. In a five-year project, Dr. James C. Wren studied 347 atherosclerotic patients—174 women and 173 men—with only 31 considered clinically hypothyroid or with lab values below the normal range. With this in mind, all patients were given thyroid supplementation, and results were then calculated. Many of the patients experienced significant improvement and their mortality rate was cut in half of what is usual for this type of untreated patient. What is truly amazing about this study is that only *nine* percent had diagnosed hypothyroidism, yet a majority of participants reaped benefits from their thyroid supplementation. You'll understand this discrepancy more thoroughly throughout the rest of the chapter.

Throughout this book, I have expressed every hormone's absolute importance and necessity, but the thyroid is especially vital since it affects every organ, cell, and hormone in the body. The body cannot survive without its presence, and when it's even mildly deficient, the body can suffer from high cholesterol and triglyceride levels, sluggish thought processes and memory, sexual dysfunction, weight gain, and osteoporosis. Since the symptomatic spectrum is vast, doctors have a hard time putting their finger on the thyroid as the culprit, and many times, patients are shuffled from one doctor to the next or one medication to another. Insufficient-thyroid-induced depression may be treated with an anti-depressant, or hypothyroid-influenced weight gain may be attributed to a poor diet and exercise regimen. When a person is suffering from hypothyroidism or insufficient thyroid levels, an anti-depressant, or a low-fat diet/high-caliber exercise program is basically a waste of time. In spite of "normal" thyroid levels on standard blood tests, results are only seen with the restoration of the thyroid to optimal levels.

Along with the thyroid enigma, there is the controversy that surrounds what kind of thyroid should be used in treating patients. Some doctors believe that the "pure" form, or Synthroid, works the best, while other doctors are emphatically in the natural, desiccated Armour Thyroid camp. I happen to sit firmly in the latter. I will discuss this heated debate later on in the chapter, along with the differences of the two kinds of hormones and why I, along with many of my forward-thinking colleagues, choose Armour Thyroid. It raises the active thyroid hormone called T3, while synthroid and other synthetic T4 preparations do not.

To understand the mystery behind the thyroid, and whether or not you suffer from hypothyroidism or an age-related decline in thyroid levels, I think it is imperative for you to have a clear understanding of its capabilities at optimal levels and what havoc it causes when it dips below normal levels or settles at low-normal ranges (where many patients with symptoms reside).

Your Amazing Thyroid

Your thyroid is the butterfly shaped gland that wraps around the front of your windpipe. It varies in weight, but is usually about one ounce. Fascinatingly enough, the thyroid gland only secretes a tablespoon of this metabolic hormone a year and a majority of it is bound to a protein, making it useless to tissues. Yet, that seemingly insignificant amount makes a world of difference to your body. It is critical to the growth, differentiation, and metabolism of each cell in the body. It regulates temperature, metabolism, and cerebral function. It increases breakdown of fat and lowers cholesterol levels, protecting you against heart disease. This amazing hormone increases your cerebral metabolism and prevents cognitive decline. Without an optimal amount of thyroid, people might suffer from a range of complications: lethargy, forgetfulness, mental confusion, depression, arthritis-like pain, and a susceptibility to being cold and catching colds.

There are actually two types of hormones that the thyroid secretes: thyroxine, also known as T4, and triiodothyronine, known as T3. About 80 percent of the thyroid we produce is T4, the weaker thyroid hormone, while T3, the active hormone, makes up only about 20 percent of the thyroid, yet is four times stronger than T4. These hormones are composed of the amino acid tyrosine, obtained from dietary protein, and contain four and three iodine atoms respectively.

The liver and other tissues convert T4 to T3 to achieve maximum cellular effectiveness. The secretion of these two hormones is stimulated by the pituitary gland's secretion of thyroid-stimulating hormone (TSH), which is regulated by a substance secreted by the hypothalamus called thyroid-stimulating hormone releasing factor (TRF). It's a long chain of events to get that small, yet key ingredient for optimal health.

When an inefficient supply of thyroid is caused by a malfunction in the gland itself, it is called primary hypothyroidism. High TSH levels usually indicate this, since the pituitary can still sense a drop in thyroid. When under-production is caused by either the hypothalamus or the pituitary gland, it is called secondary hypothyroidism. This is indicated by low TSH, which halts the production of T4 and T3. Both problems are usually reconciled with thyroid supplementation. Another, yet controversial, reason for thyroid reduction is an age-related insensitivity of the receptor sites. I say controversial because many endocrinologists as well as other doctors refuse to believe that the receptor sites become desensitized with aging. Yet, there are times when patients have all the symptoms of a hypothyroid patient, but the outcome of their thyroid tests are normal. These patients are usually left to fend for themselves because the numbers do not reflect a thyroid insufficiency, and unfortunately, many doctors opt to treat the numbers, rather than the symptoms. However, if thyroid is prescribed, the doctor will notice that the symptoms reduce, giving credence to the thyroid resistance or receptor insensitivity theory.

Another biological problem, just recently uncovered, is a third type of thyroid, which has proved to be rather a transposed-thyroid. It usually kicks in when a person experiences such extreme circumstances as famine, or self-imposed fasting. This can also happen because people lack the proper enzymes, preventing the ideal conversion into T3. In normal settings, our thyroid works to ensure an efficient utilization of energy, but in such conditions as stated above, T4 converts into a reverse T3. This rT3 impersonates or masquerades as T3 so well that it binds to thyroid receptors in cells, making them inaccessible to normal T3. This lowers the body temperature, decreases energy production, and causes an overall physical and mental sluggishness. In times of famine, this metabolic slowing saves lives. But sometimes a diet can trigger rT3 production, causing the exact opposite results than desired: severe weight gain and fatigue. Not only does a strict diet contribute to the production of rT3, but it is also age-influenced and stress-influenced. Age and stress may also coincide, eliciting a condition that can become permanent, and thereby the body has a difficult time returning to a normal thyroid balance.

Since the thyroid still makes T4, which converts into T3 along with its doppelganger rT3, the TSH remains normal and blood tests fool doctors into not suspecting the thyroid. One way of getting around this is explained in the next section, taking your basal body temperature several times a day.

Before moving on to the next segment, I must warn you that finding a doctor aware of the above problem is rare. It is hard enough to be diagnosed with normal hypothyroidism, so you can imagine how hard it would be for a doctor to relate to a possible reverse T3 difficulty. Also, many doctors remain naïve to testing for low free T3 levels, and therefore never equate low T3 levels with the signature symptoms of thyroid insufficiency. If the TSH and T4 levels are normal, then your symptoms lack a thyroid basis to your argument. It's up to you to become aware of the possibilities and present them to your doctor. If your doctor is still unconvinced, search out one that will listen. It is your body, and perhaps you're more aware than a doctor exactly what it needs and what it can do without.

Cold to the Touch

A good question to ask yourself is whether or not you feel cold to the touch. Whether or not people comment that your hands are cold as ice, or it seems no matter how many blankets you pile on your feet, they never seem to feel warm enough. Does this sound familiar? To many people it does. You're freezing in your office while the lady across the hall just took off her sweater. This is actually one of the telltale signs of thyroid insufficiency—which also led to probably the most simple and inexpensive tests for hypothyroidism: taking your temperature.

Dr. Broda O. Barnes, a long time proponent, and perhaps the godfather of thyroid replacement therapy, discovered that many patients who exhibited a myriad of the classical symptoms of hypothyroidism had a lower basal body temperature than people who had no complaints at all. In his revolutionizing book, <u>Hypothyroidism: The Unsuspecting Illness</u>, he illustrated a technique for detecting this illusive disease that caused fatigue, headaches, and weight problems by simply having the patient record their basal temperature for two consecutive mornings. If the temperature was low, then the patient was likely to be hypothyroid. He proved this theory, through a series of tests that indicated patients with low basal temperatures had symptoms of hypothyroidism. These symptoms lessened or disappeared with the supplementation of desiccated thyroid.

Although taking your temperature in the A.M. (I believe, for accuracy, it should also be taken in the afternoon) for four consecutive days can help to establish or confirm the symptoms you have, I don't advocate that basal body temperature be the sole provider of a hypothyroid diagnosis. There are other contingencies that can factor into a low basal temperature. Depression, stress, or eating disorders can lower the body's temperature and should be taken into consideration by yourself and your health care provider when trying to understand the cause of certain symptoms. Depression can survive outside of hypothyroidism and common mood disorders should not be treated with thyroid, unless other symptoms of hypothyroidism are obvious, as well as positive indication from TSH and free T3 and T4 blood tests. There is a delicate thyroid balance that must be attained for proper emotional and physical health.

One of my patients—we'll call her "Deana"—had lived for several years feeling, as she put it, "chilled to the bone." "I feel as if the cold actually sits in my bones and seeps from the inside out, rather than the other way around." She had been to her general practitioner, who had checked her TSH level and found it to be normal. Instead of treating the symptoms, he simply treated the blood test and sent her on her way empty-handed. When she came to see me with another problem, she mentioned how cold she felt all the time. "I live in Southern California, and I feel as if I'm at the North Pole. I'm freezing." Deana was also tired quite often and fell into unexplainable lows throughout the day. She frequently felt drained of energy. "Even if I get a good solid eight hours of sleep, I still can't keep my eyes open."

She was surprised at my interest in her story, as she was used to this abnormality as a fact of life. We tested her free T3 levels and found that she was low-grade hypothyroid. After a month of thyroid supplementation her thyroid levels went back to normal. Deana had a stable level of energy throughout the day and she didn't have to wear a sweater to work anymore. She called to say, "So this is what Southern California feels like." She also gushed about how her thin skin, hair, and nails were improving.

Temperature is basically dependent on the metabolic process, which is governed by optimal thyroid levels. If your temperature dips below normal, the pituitary gland increases TSH production, which in turn, provokes a production of thyroid. In this way the body generates the heat to offset cold temperatures. When thyroid levels dip, so does our body's temperature. When our temperatures go even a degree above or below 98.6, the effects are felt immediately. This slower metabolic process can cause havoc on many systems we take for granted. We actually start experiencing sluggish movement and slower speech. Our thought processes also slows down, and we experience lapses in short-term memory. Even our bone marrow suffers when our bodies are at lower temperatures. Bone marrow is responsible for the production of red blood cells, which circulate oxygen throughout the body, and white blood cells, which work to protect the body against bacteria and infection. Also, the difficulty in producing red blood cells can cause other problems, like anemia. Anemia factors into fatigue, and fatigue factors into depression. It seems the symptoms of hypothyroidism are interrelated, one tag-teaming the other. Many times, patients with hypothyroidism will not only be cold, but without the help of red and white blood cells, these patients also suffer from a variety of colds and flues.

At optimal levels, the thyroid regulates the body's temperature, which manages important processes like the workings of the immune system and our cerebral functioning. When our bodies are at the right temperature, 98.6 degrees, they are able to work efficiently: the immune system can block illnesses, physical movement is faster, and mental processes, like memory, work properly. Normal temperatures are essential for enzyme functioning and preservation of health.

However, feeling cold is the least of your worries. Victims of hypothyroidism and low thyroid levels often find themselves feeling disconnected from the world around them. They can't keep up, nor do they want to, and they seem to fade from the dynamic and changing world around them. In the next section, you will find that perhaps your exhaustion and depression are not a way of life, but rather symptoms of a curable complication—hypothyroidism or insufficient thyroid levels.

News to Cure the Blues

"Doctor, I think I'm losing it. If I could just sleep through the rest of these years, I think I could make it." "Beverly," of course wasn't serious, but she was desperate for help. Her world had come crashing down a year ago, and since then she found herself physically and emotionally challenged. What happened? She simply became thyroid insufficient. What caused it? Well, doctors may have varying opinions, but I believe stress from a divorce and a parent's illness factored into it manifesting itself. Depression and fatigue lead the list of the most common symptoms of insufficient thyroid levels. Also these symptoms seem to go misdiagnosed or ignored for various reasons. In Beverly's case, her doctor blamed her mood swings and weariness on the strain due to her previous stressful experiences. He did the proper blood tests, which include measuring the TSH but excluding the free T3, and found no problems there. So, he loaded her up on all kinds of medications: anti-anxiety, anti-depressants, valium, and referred her to a really good psychiatrist. Think of Beverly's dismay when she realized her arsenal of medications and therapy only made her feel worse. Her doctor failed to be thorough by doing *all* the blood tests, and therefore, failed to find she was hypothyroid. To him, she was essentially an open and shut case.

Beverly is not alone. Many people, women more often than men, find themselves trapped into feeling ignored. Unfortunately, too many of them suffer a long time before they find a doctor willing to listen to the symptoms, do the proper tests, and consider the two together when making a prognosis. I think, especially when it comes to something as illusive as hypothyroidism or low-normal thyroid levels, doctors become lazy and rely exclusively on blood tests. If the blood tests reveal no abnormality, then the patient is healthy and the symptoms are merely dismissed as psychosomatic. I believe before the tests, a doctor must listen to the symptoms and treat the patient. The tests should be looked upon as information that can allow the doctor to more thoroughly understand and minister to the problem. My dictum is any depression, fatigue, or symptoms of feeling lousy are due to thyroid deficiency, unless proven otherwise. I also should add that testing for thyroid malfunction is a great way to rule out depression and manic-depression. There is no reason to treat a depression that isn't really there. What is truly frightening is that some forms of medication used for depression can cause more damage than good. Lithium, which is used to treat unipolar or bipolar depression, might actually cause or worsen hypothyroidism. This is why it is vitally important for doctors to be absolutely certain the source of the depression and how to treat it.

In a study reported in the *Archives of General Psychiatry*, ten out of the eleven patients experienced notable improvement in depressive symptoms when high doses of thyroid medication were added to their current medicinal regimens. Five out of seven of the patients also encountered relief of manic symptoms with the addition of thyroid. The administrators of the study suggested that perhaps depression disorders as seen in rapid cycling and other refractory affective disorders may be due to a deficit in brain thyroid hormone. They theorized that adequate amounts of thyroid were not reaching the brain or not being processed correctly, even though most of the patients had normal circulating levels of thyroid hormones.

After a year of battling with her sub-clinical depression, Beverly started researching depression on the Internet. She stumbled upon thyroid deficiency and recognized her symptoms as classic. When she approached her doctor, he grudgingly tested her TSH levels, which were found to be in the normal range. She was at a dead end. One of her co-workers, who believed she was menopausal, referred her to me. Through tears, she explained her symptoms. "I'm either sad, apathetic, or just plain worn out. I'm basically flattened by whatever it is that's working me over." I tested her TSH and free T3 levels and found that although her TSH was normal, her T3 ranged quite low. She was definitely lacking the essential feel-good hormone. Within months of supplementation of desiccated Armour thyroid, she felt the vitality she once experienced before her father's illness and her divorce. She again felt empowered and in control of how she felt and acted.

Mary Shoman, a long time researcher on thyroid insufficiency, administered a poll at a thyroid forum. She asked people what they felt were the worst symptoms of thyroid disease. Over seven hundred people answered the poll and twenty-three percent believed their related depression problems were the hardest to cope with.

The thyroid plays a large role in our physical well-being as well as how we emotionally perceive the world around us. When the thyroid is at proper levels, stressful events are handled with ease and fatigue is not a common, unexplainable occurrence. If thyroid levels dip, fatigue, depression, mood swings, and sluggish thought processes—although not considered clinically "psychiatric"—can seriously hamper a patient's lifestyle and peace of mind.

According to the Thyroid Society:

> Most patients with hypothyroidism have some degree of associated depression, ranging from mild to severe. 10 percent to 15 percent of the patients with a diagnosis of depression may have thyroid deficiency. Patients with depression should be tested to determine if they have a thyroid disorder.
> Several research studies have been done and continue to be done on the association between depression and thyroid disease. Although all forms of depression, including bipolar disorders like manic depression, can be found in either hypothyroidism or hyperthyroidism, depression is more often associated with hypothyroidism.

Subclinical hypothyroidism can also manifest some serious symptoms. What we take for granted—our good mood and humor, our ability to get through the day without nodding off, or our ability to remember so and so's birthday—suddenly become monumental tasks. We're being incapacitated by the one gland we have unknowingly been dependent on for years, the thyroid gland.

Psychiatrists often describe depression as "something chemically wrong." They're really not too far from the truth. A patient who is thyroid deficient is missing the all-essential chemical make-up of the thyroid hormone. Because the thyroid regulates the metabolism and influences most major organs in your body, like your heart, brain, kidneys, liver, ovaries and testicles, along with muscles and skin, it is no wonder that many thyroid patients feel despondent and unhappy. Insufficient thyroid levels cause havoc on many components of the body and mind, and a good many of those components effect how you feel about yourself. With an underactive thyroid, skin becomes dry, nails become brittle, hair thins, pounds accumulate, and a person often feels tired and on the edge. All this adds up into depression. And whether it is subclinical or full-blown depression, your body is essentially reacting to the absence of thyroid.

Even when a patient's hypothyroidism or low thyroid levels have been detected, most patients are prescribed the wrong kind of thyroid. Such is the case of one of my patients, "Janet", who had been diagnosed hypothyroid and treated with Synthroid over a year's span. She described this time in her life as gloomy and unsettled. "I felt like I couldn't cope with the simplest of issues, like the garbage disposal not working or a shoelace breaking. I would cry for no apparent reason. It was worse than when I went through menopause." Basically, although her hypothyroidism had been treated, Janet was essentially still hypothyroid. When she sought me out through a suggestion of a friend, I listened to her story and simply let her know she was on the wrong thyroid medication. I showed her an article from the *New England Journal of Medicine* (which I will discuss later on in the chapter) that explained that many times patients have more success and feel better faster if they are supplemented with a natural thyroid. I gave her a prescription of Armour thyroid and asked her to call me in a few weeks. When she called, she had nothing but positive things to say. "I feel alive again. My husband isn't walking on eggshells anymore and I feel like I can finally breathe freely. It's amazing."

The lack of sufficient thyroid levels can also make thinking clearly virtually impossible. Patients complain they're tired and their minds are cloudy with fatigue. This cognitive haze is actually not uncommon. In a 1999 article entitled, *Thyroid Hormones: Positive Relationships with Cognition in Healthy Euthyroid Older Men*, the subjects on a middle to high combination of T4/T3 were able to maintain high brain functioning. This study confirmed the method of supplementing thyroid even when studies designate the patient is not in need of thyroid. The results in this study suggest that older men (and older women) with low normal T4 levels may benefit cognitively from thyroid supplementation. Yet, even in light of these findings, many doctors lack the confidence in supplementing thyroid without blood tests to support the action. I believe doctors' motives should be to increase the well-being of their patients and not worry so much about lab tests, and as you can see, contemporary studies in some of our best medical journals are coming around to the same methods of medicine.

What I find amazing is that first, patients with symptoms of depression are never checked for thyroid dysfunction. And second, if their hypothyroidism is detected they are given a hormone supplement that will not supply them with adequate thyroid levels and therefore, their symptomatic depression rarely subsides. If you suffer from depression and you haven't found the source or a veritable cure, you may be suffering from insufficient thyroid levels. Depression is a debilitating disease that affects your ability to think clearly and act promptly. With the help of thyroid supplementation, your symptoms will become a past topic, allowing you to focus on a limitless future. Study after study shows that even patients with normal TSH levels feel better on a combination of T4 and T3 therapy. I encourage you to allow this information to motivate you to break free from the bonds of depression and find a future without the blues.

Weak From Fatigue?

In Mary Shoman's survey I mentioned in the previous segment, fatigue and exhaustion received the highest votes (237 out of 70, 34%) for the hardest symptom to contend with in hypothyroid sufferers. You get a good night's rest but your days are filled with a vexing sluggishness. When your metabolic rate slows down, you slow down. Fatigue makes people react in a wide array of ways. Some people are tense and irritable, while others become despondent and withdrawn from social situations. Other symptoms of hypothyroidism only contribute to fatigue. Anemia, slowing of the heartbeat, headaches, and emotional disorders all leave a person feeling drained and overworked.

Doctors across America record over 500 million patient visits in regards to fatigue, and the sad thing is that rarely do patients find a cure and being tired has become as familiar to them as breathing. The complaint of fatigue is baffling to many doctors who sidestep the source by recommending more exercise, a better diet, and more sleep. All good advice, yet the patient is no closer to discovering the root or origin of the problem and therefore, no closer to finding a cure. If a person is hypothyroid or simply suffering from low levels of thyroid, I can guarantee that a good diet and exercise program doubled with eight hours of sleep will not eliminate the exhaustion.

Studies have shown, as well as my own observations in my patients, that the supplementation of a natural thyroid T4/T3 combination will provide the desired results—no more fatigue. Fatigue is not a normal part of your hectic life, nor is it a typical aspect of growing old. I had a patient, who, at the age of sixty-one, was told to "get over it—weariness and aging go hand in hand." Luckily, she didn't "get over it" and instead she located me and I let her know that aging and fatigue were no more related than the Pope is to Buddha. She laughed with relief. I put her on Armour thyroid and within weeks she was playing golf with her husband and tending her grandkids. As a culture, we have come to accept and expect to experience the stereotypical representation of aging: slow speech, listlessness, forgetfulness, and irritability. I don't know about you, but that is nothing to look forward to. Fatigue, like depression, weight gain, and intolerance to cold temperatures can be lessened, if not cured, with the proper supplementation of thyroid. The cure is easy. Finding a doctor willing to prescribe you the cure is the hard part. Feeling better and reclaiming your active lifestyle should be enough reason to spur you on in your pursuit of finding a doctor willing to be your partner in your wellness and longevity. I guarantee that the time will be well spent when you can work throughout an entire day without nodding off or guzzling five cups of coffee to just get you through the next few hours. Once you are on the right type of thyroid at the correct dose you will notice a world of difference.

Symptoms are not the only reason to look into a yearly thyroid check-up. Your heart as well as other internal organs, that are not so overt about letting you in on their optimal well-being, also suffer the consequences of thyroid dysfunction. As you will discover in the next segment, your heart and your thyroid gland are inseparable as far as your longevity is concerned.

Thyroid for the Heart?

Certain hormones are known for their heart healthy contributions. Estrogen has been proven, without a doubt, to limit the incidence of heart disease and stroke. Testosterone, in turn, guards a man from possibly knowing what it feels like to be rushed to the emergency room from fear-influenced angina pains. But, what about the thyroid? Where does it fit into the heart-healthy equation? As far as cholesterol, weight gain, and increased blood pressure is concerned, the thyroid is one the forefront leaders in heart disease prevention. Because the thyroid is in charge of the metabolic process, and because metabolism and energy supply depend upon optimal levels of thyroid, it seems safe to say, the heart's health depends heavily on thyroid function.

The thyroid hormone indirectly and directly influences the health of the cardiovascular system, and whether it is a thyroid dysfunction that alters the heart's health or it is a cardiovascular disease that hampers the thyroid function, it's evident that the two are closely related and are interdependent on each other. Doctors and researchers alike have found through invasive and noninvasive procedures that thyroid status affects heart rate, cardiac output, and systemic vascular resistance. Groundbreaking studies are now finding that many aspects of heart disease are closely related to thyroid dysfunction. Hypothyroidism, in particular, whether overt or merely subclinical, causes hypertension or high blood pressure, a narrowed pulse pressure, and high serum concentrations of cholesterol.

Other findings have shown that hypothyroidism is directly linked to elevated homocysteine levels, the amino acid considered a risk factor for vascular occlusion, and these elevated levels may be an independent indicator for atherosclerosis (hardening of the arteries). In a 1999 study, researchers from the Cleveland Clinic observed how thyroid replacement therapy influenced the homocysteine levels in hypothyroid patients. All four hypothyroid men and four of the ten hypothyroid women had high homocysteine levels, compared to levels of healthy volunteer men and women. After administration, the thyroid levels returned to normal and seven of the eight patients had a significant drop in homocysteine levels. This is an exciting study since it indicates that hypothyroidism may be a treatable cause of hyperhomocysteinemia. As shown above, the thyroid supplementation returned the homocysteine levels to normal, and thereby lowered the possible risk of atherosclerosis.

Other studies have approached the subject of subclinical hypothyroidism, and although means of treating this problem are a subject of disagreement among doctors, one thing is certain, it is dangerous to the heart, and if untreated it can become overt and motivate worse cardiovascular problems. One of the big problems with subclinical hypothyroidism is that many times patients do not experience the physical and obvious symptoms of hypothyroidism. Their lives are not always afflicted by depression, intolerance to cold, low metabolism, dry skin, or mental and physical lethargy, but their hearts still suffer from this altered thyroid status. They have an increase in cholesterol and blood pressure, along with hardened arteries. The Rotterdam Study focused on the effects of subclinical hypothyroidism and discovered about 10.8 % of women in their sixties and seventies suffer from this form of hypothyroidism. Through this grand scale study completed in the Netherlands of 1149 postmenopausal women, they were able to show that the women with subclinical hypothyroidism had a more likely chance to have a history of myocardial infarction and had a higher frequency of calcification of the aorta. Therefore, the researchers determined that the women with subclinical hypothyroidism had twice as likely a chance of suffering from aortic atherosclerosis and myocardial infarction. This is important to understand since many times thyroid testing only takes place when someone is motivated to see a doctor over nagging symptoms that refuse to go away. Sometimes, in subclinical hypothyroidism, there are no symptoms to indicate a thyroid dysfunction, and therefore doctors fail to check and see if a thyroid insufficiency could be the culprit behind the heart disease risks. This is extremely important, as I'll explain later in this segment, since thyroid replacement can lessen or *eliminate* the risk of heart disease.

With this in mind, it is nice to know that some national associations are recommending that doctors include thyroid screenings in their check-up regimen. New guidelines from the American Thyroid Association states that everyone should be screened for thyroid problems as early as age thirty-five and that they should continue to screen thereon every five years. Patients with overt symptoms should be checked at more regular intervals. Being a doctor who understands that patients, as they get older, have an increased chance of thyroid dysfunction, it's refreshing to see that others are also beginning to understand the necessity of optimal thyroid levels. The American College of Physicians has also recommended thyroid screening for women over fifty for several years.

Many studies have shown that when patients at risk for heart disease are supplemented with both forms of thyroid, the T4 and T3, they experience positive results. Studies have proven thyroid therapy can reverse *all* the cardiovascular alterations influenced by hypothyroidism. A large study of patients with hypothyroidism and clinical evidence of ischemic heart disease showed significant results with the initiation of thyroid hormone therapy. New or worsening angina pains or acute myocardial infarction was rare. This study only emphasized what other studies have found: thyroid hormone supplementation improves the efficiency of myocardial oxygen consumption and lowers systemic vascular resistance.

Another study on thyroid replacement yielded still more positive results in twenty patients. When treated with thyroxine daily for twelve weeks, the patients' exercise performance improved dramatically, and their ability to reach optimal heartbeats per minute while exercising increased while their systemic blood flow resistance decreased.

Heart failure is still the number one killer in the United States for both men and women. Doctors and researchers have been prying the heart, so to speak, to find out the different faces of cardiovascular disease. One of these faces is thyroid insufficiency. In patients with uncomplicated acute myocardial infarction (a part of the heart dies due to insufficient blood flow), serum triiodothyronine (T3) levels fell by about 20 percent, while free serum triiodothyronine levels dropped an *entire* 40 percent. However, here is good news and hope for patients with acute chronic cardiac disease. Since T3 works at the cellular level, it affects cardiac myocites (cardiac muscle cells). Many studies have found that triiodothyronine is a big proponent of vasodilation, since it affects the vascular smooth-muscle cells that promote relaxation. Doctors have discovered that it significantly increases cardiac output, just hours after coronary-artery bypass grafting. This is extremely revealing information in light of the delicate post-surgery setting for the heart.

Other studies have revealed T3's awesome restoration power. In an analysis of twenty-three patients with advanced heart failure, a single intravenous dose of T3 resulted in an increase of cardiac output and a decrease in resistance of blood in the circulatory system only *two* hours after administration, without any negative effects, like rhythm disturbances.

T3 and T4 have a stunning and fascinating relationship with the cardiovascular system. Study after study confirms that they go hand in hand in ensuring your health. The clinical cases above are worst-case scenarios but I cited them to give you some idea of the kind of powerful influence the thyroid has over the heart. It pumps out our life source, and as we age, the pumping becomes more difficult and blood flow encounters obstacles. Thyroid inhibits those obstacles and difficulties from happening. The thyroid is truly a dynamic hormone that seems to have a hand in all the important processes of the body and mind and that is why I cannot stress enough the absolute necessity to make thyroid testing, (both TSH levels and free T3 and T4 levels) a part of your yearly check-up regimen. Find a doctor open to giving full attention to your thyroid health; your heart will be healthier for it and the years ahead will be unhampered by fears of heart disease.

I'm in the Normal Range, but I Feel Terrible.

How many of you have actually been diagnosed with hypothyroidism, and you let go a sigh of relief because there was a reason behind the fatigue, depression, absentmindedness, and weight gain. Your doctor prescribed you the most popular cure, Synthroid, and sent you on your way. Do you feel better? Or how many of you have normal blood tests (TSH/T4) but you've read countless articles and books on hypothyroidism and recognize yourself in many of the symptom descriptions? Many times I treat patients who have been labeled "normal." Their TSH and T4 tests are normal and all systems, except for their symptoms, check out "O.K." Their doctors can't seem to reconcile themselves to prescribing thyroid merely for unsubstantiated or unfounded symptoms. So, their symptoms remain cureless or a figment of their imagination.

Mary Shoman, the thyroid guru for the layman, refers to this pandemic of overlooked symptoms as "undertreated hypothyroidism." She defines it as hypothyroidism on a cellular level, which means, although the TSH level remains "normal," the patient still suffers from such symptoms as fatigue, weight gain, depression, muscle/joint pain, and hair and skin dryness. This can happen for many reasons: the wrong medicine (Synthroid) or the wrong estimation of what TSH levels are "normal." *The British Medical Journal* has new information and research that may disprove the theory by many doctors, general practitioners and endocrinologists alike, that states a TSH level of one to two is normal. The journal suggests that values of two may prove to be abnormal.

TSH levels can indicate an illness or a deficiency some of the time, but too many doctors base their diagnosis on this alone. I firmly believe in the importance of tests measuring free T3, as well as free T4. T4 levels will not always tell the truth of thyroid insufficiency, nor will TSH. I have found that a combination of the three blood tests delivers the most accurate information in regards to thyroid health. It is important to require of your doctor to not only look at TSH, but to also take a look at the free levels of T4 and T3. TSH is an indication of the body's sensing of the total amount of thyroid, and most of that is bound to proteins, disabling it from connecting with the receptors for optimal hormonal activity.

E. Denis Wilson, MD, explains in his book Wilson's Syndrome, the theory that there is a fine, but distinct, line between thyroid gland dysfunction and thyroid system dysfunction. He believed that, on a cellular level, only T3 is effective, and although TSH and T4 levels remain normal, the all-important T3 remains deficient. I agree with Dr. Wilson to some extent, although his views are a little too T3 extreme. Unlike conventional doctors, he believes in solely a T3 preparation, based on symptoms and basal body temperature rather than blood tests. There are several flaws here. First, administering only T3 does not mimic the body's natural production of thyroid. Although T3 is the active hormone, T4's presence is also necessary. Second, basing your prognosis entirely on symptoms and temperature can get kind of sticky. As I have stated before, depression can be by itself a disease not tied to thyroid insufficiency. Depression can also alter basal body temperature. It's important that your doctor take a few things into consideration—blood tests and symptoms should both be evaluated to make a diagnosis of disease, otherwise, it's just a lot of guess work.

The best way to try to convince your doctor of your condition is to arm yourself with information regarding the disease as well as information about age related thyroid deficiency. This may prove difficult since many doctors are unaware of the tremendous health and feel-good benefits associated with thyroid replacement. I'm trying to alter this trend by lecturing to medical academies all over the United States. Also, keep a log of how you feel, perhaps create a hypothyroid checklist and check what symptoms are appropriate. Your doctor may have labeled you as "normal" but you are the only one who knows how you feel. Don't be led to believe your symptoms are psychosomatic, or that you have no basis for feeling this way. Talk to your doctor about checking your free T3 levels and other medicinal options that include a preparation of T3. If your doctor won't consider putting you on a T4/T3 therapy and refuses to listen to you, you can change your mind and your choice of physician. Your doctor should be an *active* partner in your wellness regimen.

What Thyroid Should I Be Taking?

This is where the heated debate arises, and where I disagree with many of the doctors treating thyroid complications today. I believe the crux of natural hormone replacement therapy solely resides in the hormones supplemented being exact replicates of what the body naturally makes. This is essential for the body to achieve optimal results when participating in a hormone replacement regimen. Too often, as I stated before in previous chapters, doctors are sold on one idea and one form of hormone replacement, which is usually a synthetic form pharmaceutical companies push for financial incentives. Just as you saw this mindset toward progesterone and estrogen, the same goes for thyroid.

I clarified at the beginning of this chapter that the body naturally responds to two types of thyroid, T4 and T3. And as I illustrated in the segment previous to this one, without the optimal response from both kinds of thyroid, the body cannot react properly or effectively. The optimization of metabolism and energy production through thyroid supplementation can not be emphasized enough, and although many doctors would agree with this desire of optimal wellness, the way they seek to achieve maximum metabolism or energy is all wrong.

The most popular thyroid on the market today is a product called Synthroid or its generic versions, Levoxyl or Levothroid (levothyroxine). Both only contain T4, the weaker counterpart of the thyroid, with the assumption that T4 will convert into active T3. The pharmaceutical company as well as the physicians that prescribe it would also argue that the synthetic form offers a more steady, controllable hormonal level. The problem that I've found with this theory is the T4 in Synthroid does not readily convert into T3 and although the TSH remains at a normal level and T4 levels continue to stay where they should, many patients still complain of the classic symptoms of hypothyroidism. Yet, if their doctors were to measure these patients' free T3 levels, they would be surprised to find that most likely they are quite low.

In 1996, a group of researchers made important observations in rats that they believed would be relevant and noteworthy in humans. These researchers surgically induced hypothyroidism by removing the thyroid from the rats. They found that the only way to achieve normal serum concentrations of thyroxine, triiodothyronine, and thyrotropin and tissue euthyroidism was through the administration of desiccated T4/T3 combination. When the rats were administered thyroxine alone, the researchers found that normal concentrations of the active triiodothyronine could not be reached in certain vital tissues like the liver or kidney. Therefore, the rats remained hypothyroid in many aspects of their physiology.

The battle between these two drugs, and the two camps of doctors who prescribe them, actually came to head only a few years ago. The prestigious medical journal, the *New England Journal of Medicine* reported that indeed, a combination of both T4 and T3, like found in Armour Thyroid, is more capable in treating hypothyroidism than is Synthroid. In this study, researchers observed 33 hypothyroid patients either on thyroxine (T4) alone, or on a combination of thyroxine and triiodothyronine (T4). Each patient was studied for two five-week periods; one segment of time was allotted for T4 alone, while the other for the T4/T3 combination. They found a vast improvement in mood and neuropsychological functioning in the group supplemented with both T3 and T4, rather than just Synthroid or a generic T4: "treatment with thyroxine plus triiodothyronine improved the quality of life of most patients."

The theory behind the above results was that the tissues in need of thyroid were not always capable of converting the T4 into the active T3. The researchers assessed the above statement by allotting the two groups a battery of language, learning and memory tests. The patients supplemented with the combination thyroid had higher scores than did the Synthroid group in tests measuring cognitive performance, mood, and physical status. This improvement was significant during the time the patients were on the T4/T3 combination.

The history of Armour thyroid is a long one. It has been used for centuries, really as early as 1892, and for the longest time it was the only form of therapy for hypothyroidism. But since T3 has a potent half-life, doctors shied away from its erratic nature and chose instead the "safer and controllable" T4. Synthroid became the "in" thyroid, and since it was backed by a large and profitable pharmaceutical company, studies were done in its favor. In the meantime, Armour thyroid lost its significance and doctors referred to it as "outdated."

Ever since Synthroid hit the mainstream market, I've noticed many patients fighting with a thyroid deficiency that has been supposedly cured. They take Synthroid religiously every morning, but, sadly, the best relief they can truly hope for is a placebo effect. The FDA actually fined Knoll Pharmaceutics 90 million dollars for forging results of studies, while withholding truthful but disastrous results from other studies, to convince physicians and therefore patients that Synthroid was better than the outdated Armour thyroid. I myself, along with my esteemed colleague, Dr. Douglas E. Greer, assessed the above claims in our own study of patients with normal TSH levels, some on Synthroid and some not. All had the classic symptoms of hypothyroidism: decreased energy, hair and skin changes, and slower thought processes. In our two clinical studies, we came to the conclusion that T4 alone, as seen in products like Synthroid, does not adequately convert into T3 and cannot, consequently, result in symptomatic improvement.

The first study evaluated 671 patients for about a year and a half for thyroid disease. All patients had symptoms of some thyroid insufficiency and were tested for TSH and free T4 and T3. As a part of the test, the patients were advised to take their basal body temperature. None of the patients were on any kind of thyroid therapy and the thyroid deficient symptoms were assessed to eliminate patients with problems that may be tied to another illness (i.e. depression). Many patients had low and low-normal T3 levels: 262 patients had abnormally low free T3 levels, while the rest were within the normal range, albeit, borderline normal. All had basal body temperatures of 97 degrees or less. When we added a thyroid T4/T3 supplement, their low temperatures were corrected along with the patients' sense of well-being, the normal patient response being, "I have known for years that I was hypothyroid but I have never been able to find a doctor willing to listen to me and treat me appropriately." Needless to say, we did.

The patients above were essentially ignored before our test because the conventional test, the measure of TSH, reflected a normal thyroid function. Many doctors believe that the TSH is the end all and be all of thyroid testing. If they do perceive a glitch they take care of it through T4 administration with the belief that it will eliminate any thyroid functional problems. As I will show you in the next clinical test, it will not.

We evaluated thirty-one patients (twenty-nine females and two males) presently supplemented with a T4 preparation (Synthroid or Levoxyl) to get an understanding of their bodies' compliance with T4 alone. We ordered the standard TSH lab, along with free T4 and free T3. Our data confirmed that free T3 levels were often low or sub therapeutic. No matter the amount of T4 supplemented, only the TSH levels were affected. The T3 levels, the active thyroid, remained low. This is interesting, in light of the fact that a T4 preparation is widely accepted in treating hypothyroidism. Our data flies in the face of this and instead indicates that T4 supplementation rarely converts into T3 adequately.

It is important to understand that as we age, thyroid insufficiency results from decreased production of T4, decreased conversion of T4 into T3, and decreased sensitivity of receptor sites; thereby, one of these three age-related thyroid complications can cause symptoms despite proper blood levels. The field of molecular biology is just now recognizing that this hypometabolic euthyroid syndrome occurs in spite of normal TSH and T4 levels. Idealistically, the enzyme 5-deiodinase removes the iodine atom from T4, transforming it into the metabolically active T3. Yet, any effect, any physical or emotional stress on the adrenals can hinder this enzyme from converting T4 to T3, the outcome being metabolic slowdown and hypothyroidism or insufficient thyroid. Some of these patients are not necessarily clinically ill; however, their condition is not optimal. As a doctor, I took an oath to do no harm. My job is to heal, and using one half of the equation does not equal the sum of excellent health. I am not here to sit on the fence of some pharmaceutical company and make decisions based on some mocked up test results. My patient's optimal well-being is my first priority, pleasing the public is my last. Synthroid rarely, if ever, converts into T3, and whether or not we trick the hypothalamus or pituitary gland into believing there is enough thyroid in the body, T3 is the true protagonist in our body's health.

How to be Heard

Simply listen to the patient. They will eventually tell you what the diagnosis is.
—A wise professor from medical school.

This is the tricky part. You see, hypothyroidism or an underactive thyroid is not always perceivable, as I have explained throughout this entire chapter, and trying to explain yourself to the conservative medical field may seem to be more trouble than it's worth—but believe me it's worth it. One of the problems is that there is no distinct guidelines or recommendations that the thyroid should be screened yearly after a certain time period. As I mentioned before, some organizations have suggested a routine thyroid check-up, but nothing has really been set in stone. Danese and co-researchers demonstrated that TSH screening every five years, starting at 35, was cost-effective because progression of overt hypothyroidism was prevented, serum cholesterol levels were reduced, and symptoms and complications were abated with early treatment of hypothyroidism. I believe it should be included in your *yearly* check-up, because a lot can happen in a five-year span.

Overall this is an undiagnosed epidemic. A new study found that thirteen million Americans might be unaware of, and therefore remain undiagnosed for, their thyroid dysfunction. The Colorado Thyroid Disease Prevalence Study took 25, 862 participants at the Colorado statewide health fair in 1995. Among people not taking thyroid, they found that 8.9 percent were hypothyroid, while 1.1 percent were hyperthyroid. They took these figures and applied them to the rest of the United States, which indicated that, nationally, there may be thirteen million Americans unaware that their symptoms are curable. I believe that more people are suffering from inadequate levels than the above study indicated. They used TSH levels solely as the marker of hypothyroidism, but I believe that if free T3 levels were included along with symptomatic complaints, the thirteen million could possibly double. You may be one of those undiagnosed numbers.

In light of the fact that hypothyroidism can cause undesired weight gain and skin texture changes, body temperature dips, fatigue and depression, and cardiac complications, I believe it is especially important for you and your doctor to become acquainted with your thyroid hormone. Preventive medicine is more cost effective, and it saves lives. Think about it, you could stop heart disease before it starts, you could maintain your active lifestyle well into you twilight years, and you could keep your mind and emotions in check. All these elemental facets of being healthy originate with the thyroid gland and are regulated throughout your life by sufficient thyroid levels. As you get older, they dip, but if kept at optimal levels, you don't have to resemble the stereotype of getting old. You don't have to slow down. Replacing your thyroid hormone to optimal levels, not just normal levels, as the more orthodox medical field would advise, but to the levels they once were in your twenties or thirties, will make a lifestyle change for the better. You'll lose those unwanted pounds, feel like making the most of your days, and internally you will be (all your related organs) much healthier. The implications of going untreated only escalate with each year, usually ending up in overt hypothyroidism. There is no reason to let it go this far. I urge you to seek out *optimal* health care that stresses preventative methods, rather than waiting for a problem to manifest itself and then taking measures to treat it. Your thyroid gland deserves the utmost attention because it influences our energy production and the efficiency of all our other vital organs. Your health makes a rather good case for a yearly check-up and it's up to you to be assertive about whether you will take a preventive approach to your long-term well-being. I myself chose the preventive approach and have never looked back.

Human Growth Hormone: The Ultimate Healing Hormone

I remember looking at myself in the mirror after six months on HGH. It was as if I had gone through a time warp. The skin on my face was tighter and the muscles in my arms and legs were more defined. I looked as good as I felt.
—Mathew, 56

I remember in horror, the flagging of my health. I had hip surgery and was bedridden for a month. My skin began to sag on my dwindling muscles and brittle bones—I felt like the amazing shrinking woman. After several months on HGH, my strength and stamina began to return. My doctor can't believe how fast I'm healing. I'm not quite the woman I used to be, but I'm well on my way.
—Helen, 67

Human Growth Hormone is the sexiest hormone of replacement therapy. We've seen it on TV and read about in magazines, and if you type it into a search engine, I'm sure you'll be surprised with all the products claiming to be HGH for a fraction of the price that true human growth hormone costs through a pharmacy. I'm sure you've also heard varying opinions. You may have heard Human Growth Hormone is the cure-all for aging and with its administration you can actually reverse the aging process—or, perhaps you've heard that it's overly priced and at a high price as far as side effects are concerned. You've probably seen HGH featured on primetime news magazines, with reporters skeptically questioning prescribing doctors and their famous patients, like Dixie Carter from *Designing Women,* or movie actors, like Nick Nolte. Just recently, Dateline interviewed Alan Mintz of Cenegenics in Las Vegas to understand more clearly why human growth hormone along with other anti-aging techniques are necessary and so expensive. Unfortunately, the media usually plays the part of "Chicken Little," forecasting only the worst possible scenarios, and therefore never really reporting the entire truth, just its negative side. In that particular news piece, only one clinical study was mentioned, the groundbreaking 1990 *New England Journal of Medicine* study that opened the door for HGH use in adults. Otherwise, everything since then seemed deliberately ignored. Yet, in this chapter, I will show you that human growth hormone replacement, in countless studies *after* the 1990 debut, has shown time and again to increase the quality of life and hinder the related diseases of aging. It increases lean body mass, while decreasing fat mass; and it increases bone density—eliminating osteoporosis. It is good news for heart disease and kidney failure and basically HGH awakens the body from its age-induced stupor.

As with all the hormonal therapies, the use of HGH is to perpetuate life without sacrificing the quality. We've seen the quintessential aged person of ninety, hunched over and broken. This prolonged example of incapacitated life is unacceptable to most people; yet even in light of the lessons we've learned from our parents and our grandparents, we still aspire to live longer. HGH administration most assuredly slows down the process of aging, in ways that other hormones cannot. Some patients have reported growth and a darkening at the roots of hair, while others have been able to pocket their reading glasses even when perusing the smallest of print. HGH truly assists with restoring the quality of life and the aspiration for longevity is no longer an unattainable hope.

In this chapter I will uncover all the benefits of human growth hormone and why I recommend its application, along with how I use it in my own practice. I believe in the merits of HGH, and I've seen it increase the quality of life and health among many of my patients.

Yet, I don't believe in *all* the hype that HGH has accumulated since 1990. In this chapter, I will also try to dispel any of the "get young quick schemes" you may have encountered on the Internet or in books regarding growth hormone replacement. I'm somewhat cautious when speaking about this hormone because other doctors and patients are not. This chapter will not be sprinkled with miracle stories, such as Lazarus awakening from the dead, nor will I speak of a one-time injection-stimulated euphoria—a bedridden patient doing cartwheels after one administration. This kind of fiction clouds the clinical relevance of HGH, and in the long run creates more problems for serious-minded doctors like myself, and a disappointment for patients seeking the fountain of youth.

Another conundrum of HGH is that it is expensive. Perhaps part of the hype over HGH is a matter of trying to sell it, or perhaps it is a result of patients shelling out a lot of money and therefore expecting to see miraculous and sudden results. I don't want to downplay the results of HGH because they are important to understand and they are amazing, but they happen over time and every patient is different and will experience varying outcomes. I stress that in my practice, taking human growth hormone is an elective therapy. It's not mandatory, and you can reap many rewards from a hormone plan that excludes growth hormone.

The reason I call HGH the healing hormone is quite simple, I've personally seen it at work. My wife, Carolyn, and I searched out growth hormone for its purported healing effects, after she had a sport's injury that wouldn't heal. I myself was beginning to feel the first inconveniences of aging and was willing to try anything to turn back the clock. Growth hormone, along with the other important hormones, mended Carolyn's nagging sport's injury and turned back time for the both of us. This is why the sports and Olympic industry is being infiltrated by the use of growth hormone. It increases muscle mass, yes, but more importantly it decreases the healing time for athletes after strenuous exercise or competition. I don't believe young men and women should hinder or destroy the natural secretion of their hormones by administering it with an outside source, yet their example paints an interesting picture for the older crowd. Not only have I seen a rapid healing in my wife, but many patients who have suffered falls or have had invasive surgery have also experienced quick recoveries. One of my patients had her thyroid removed because of cancer. Because she continued growth hormone therapy through and after the surgery, her recovery time was cut in half. Her doctor marveled at the efficiency of her body to handle this kind of surgery and remained skeptical at her claims that growth hormone did the trick.

Although I will remain cautious with this subject, I would like the reader to also understand that although the outlandish claims that human growth hormone can basically bring back the dead should be taken with a grain of salt, claims of growth hormone supplementation being linked to early mortality are just as equally false. With responsible and proper use, as with any potent hormone, human growth hormone can help achieve the longevity dream.

The History of Human Growth Hormone

Human growth hormone, or somatotropin, a single-chain peptide of 191amino acids, is the most abundant hormone in the body and is produced by the somatroph cells of the anterior pituitary gland. The hypothalamus stimulates the secretion of HGH with the production of growth hormone-releasing hormone (GH-RH) or inhibits the production by secreting somatostatin. Its secretion is pulsatile, with the largest pulse of production taking place at night—there is some truth behind the phrase, "We grow in our sleep." The binding of HGH to receptor molecules initiates a cascade of events that result in the secretion of IGF-I (insulin-like growth factor I), which mediates many of the biological actions of growth hormone. HGH is vital to almost every organ in the body for proper growth and development, thus its peak coincides when we need it the most—puberty. After this point, the body sees a gradual decline of growth hormone volume, to the extent that after thirty years of age a 14 percent drop occurs with each passing decade. This drop instigates many age-related physical declines as well as health related deteriorations. Growth hormone deficiency is marked by complaints of decreased energy, loss of sociability, irritability, and an inability to exercise or sleep. Physically speaking, patients with low growth hormone levels have thinning hair, increased wrinkles, sagging and loose skin, frail nails, decreased muscle strength and size, and increased abdominal fat. Diseases associated with HGH deficiency are cardiovascular disease, decreased renal function, hyperlipidemia and insulin resistance, osteoporosis, and decreased healing capabilities. Yet, all these complications suspiciously sound like the "normal" processes of aging. And they are. We are all subject to a significant drop in growth hormone levels. At the age of 40 our growth hormone production is 40 percent of what we produced at age 20, and its decline is attributable to many of the problems we associate as fact-of-life aging—problems, if not prevented with HRT, we will have to deal with and live through.

Many doctors and scientists are baffled by the drastic drop of growth hormone between the ages of 20-40. Aged somatroph cells can produce as much growth hormone as young somatroph cells, so some speculate that the problem lies in the GH inhibitor, somastatin, which increases with aging. Other theories that surround the decrease of growth hormone focus on a weakening of the pituitary gland's sensitivity to growth hormone-releasing hormone, while still others believe that receptor sites for growth hormone become less sensitive with aging. Whatever the theory of why growth hormone drops, the fact remains that its drop is far-reaching throughout the human body.

The 1990 study I mentioned at the beginning of the chapter opened the floodgates of interest toward the realm of anti-aging. The hormone, only used for children with stunted growth or dwarfism, found a new place in the adult domain with the release of the shocking Rudman study. This landmark study showed that growth hormone-deficient men who were administered HGH for six months experienced significant increases in lean body mass (8.8 percent), decreases in fatty tissue mass (14.4 percent), and increases in skin thickness (7.1 percent). The placebo group showed no remarkable change in any of the above areas. Rudman was quoted saying, "the effects of six months of human growth hormone on lean body mass and adipose-tissue mass were equivalent in magnitude to the changes incurred during 10-20 years of aging." The lucky test subjects basically demonstrated a 20-year age-reversal in some of the age-related changes that had accrued over the years, *in less than a year of replacement.*

With this study, adult onset of growth hormone deficiency was recognized and many people wanted to know if they fit the bill and how they could reap the benefits if they did. Yet, of course, as with all hormone replacement therapy it's not that easy.

Human Growth Hormone has had a rocky history. It was first derived from the pituitary of human cadavers beginning in 1958 and continuing into 1985. This hormone was distributed throughout the United State to treat growth complications, pituitary dwarfism, in nearly 8,000 children. Unfortunately, in 1985, three young men treated with the cadaver produced growth hormone died from Creutzfeldt-Jakob disease, akin to Mad Cow disease, a rare and incurable brain disease. Quickly, the cadaver growth hormone was removed from the market.

In the last decade, researchers and chemists devised a specialized way of genetically engineering growth hormone from bacteria. This may sound odd, and somewhat of a deterrent, but to set your mind at ease—it is the exact same procedure in which safe and effective insulin is made. This new recombinant growth hormone eliminated any contamination that was found in the earlier HGH therapy, while still enhancing the growth in children.

Yet, children were not the only testing group. Researchers were also trying their luck at the effects of growth hormone replacement in older subjects. Over the past decade, our knowledge has expanded in the cellular and molecular mechanisms involved in the action of growth hormone in adults. Studies have shown that the decrease of human growth hormone is directly associated with many attributable characteristics of aging, like cardiovascular disease, increased body fat, muscle wasting, wrinkled and dry skin, osteoporosis, decreased energy and sleep, and gray hair. Studies and patient testimonials have also shown that administration of growth hormone can reduce or reverse the biological effects of many of the above aspects of getting older.

Since the introduction of Rudman's study, growth hormone's fame has entered the arena of the media. Doctors now prescribe human growth hormone for its longevity effects and patients are enjoying their fifth through eighth decades like we've never seen the aged do before. This is truly a century of medicine to be excited about and grateful to grow up in.

Hanging Depression Out to Dry

Depression is a substantial part of aging in many people. It seems not just the very aged feel the blues, but also people in their first rites of aging begin to feel the rub of depression. It makes sense that as the body wanes so would the mood, but as I have shown you with all forms of hormone replacement, the body returns to its optimal strength as well as emotional well-being. I've seen the results of adding growth hormone to patients' hormone regimens, and I've seen its added boost to their frame of mind. In one case specifically, I remember a patient, Jonathan, a lawyer, who basically regarded life after sixty to be anticlimactic. He felt cheated on the reward he had worked so hard to achieve and his outlook on the future became dulled. He resented his body and he became mentally lazy—he felt lethargic and bored with his surroundings and life after his career. He felt spent. His "quality of life" spiraled down into a veritable depression that he couldn't shake. A new lover of his, who had been a client of mine for several years, suggested that he make an appointment with me. She assured him that this doctor wouldn't consider his aging normal, and that aging didn't have to be a phase to get used to. She claimed that after my therapy, the only adaptation he would to get used to is feeling better and younger. His first comment to me, however, was sarcastic: "They call these years the golden years?" After several blood tests, I understood better exactly what he was talking about—his levels were nothing close to be golden. His testosterone was low, his thyroid was short of optimal, and his growth hormone was also waning. I suggested a regimen of hormone replacement that would eliminate much of the age-related symptoms he had become anxious about. I explained that his depression and lethargy could become a past subject and that with optimal health, he could enjoy his retirement with the same zest he had enjoyed throughout his career.

Several months later, at his follow-up appointment, he expressed his gratitude. He told me that he hadn't really paid attention to his body until it stopped working, and suddenly when it occurred to him that he didn't want to go to the gym, that vacations sounded more like toil and sweat, and being sexually active made him cringe, he became scared and irritated. "I'm not one to give up and lie down, but this change in my body and mindset really threw me for a loop. With the help of growth hormone and testosterone, I'm able to enjoy retirement. I'm gardening and I go jogging every morning. I'm planning a trip to South America with my sweetheart, and I have no doubt I'll be able to trek to Macchu Picchu. I feel more alive *now* than I did when I was fifty." With optimal hormone replacement therapy, Jonathan avoided one of the biggest pitfalls of aging—a decreased quality of life. "Quality of life" is a broad term that refers to having a good physical, emotional, and mental outlook. Being in good health in all three realms is the definition of having an optimal quality of life.

As with other hormones, growth hormone enhances its user's quality of life, as it did with the example of Jonathan above. HGH helped him to focus on a future unencumbered by feeling old. He ate better, slept better, and basically lived life better. He experienced a full health turn-around. I believe part of the reason this happens is that people experience a drastic change in body composition—fat loss to muscle gain—and this modification enhances a person's sense of self-esteem. Many patients have claimed changes in skin and hair texture, elasticity, and vibrancy. Beyond the physical boundaries, they feel more energetic and youthful, more clearheaded, and have a heightened interest in the world around them.

Hypopituitary adults have shown to have a low psychological well-being with many reporting that they feel less energy, greater emotional troubles, more difficulties with sexual relationships, and a greater sense of social isolation than the control subjects. The kind of improved quality of life seen in Jonathan's case above has also been shown in many studies that illustrated the various alterations caused by HGH supplementation. In a 1997 study, psychological assessments were performed by using the well-established, independent, validated quality of life questionnaires, Nottingham Health Profile and the Psychological General Well-Being Schedule. Patients on growth hormone experienced an increased quality of life on both parameters. Other studies have illustrated the same feel-good benefits of growth hormone. *Clinical Endocrinology* reported that in two years of replacement with growth hormone, patients experienced a progressive improvement on the Nottingham Health Profile, especially in energy, emotions, and sleep. Number of sick days continued to decrease starting at six months from 12 days to seven to basically no sick days after 24 months. (This could be an incentive for bosses all over the United States.) Likewise, trips to the hospital declined from 14.9 to 7 percent after six months and remained at this level thereafter.

A study of 25 patients with adult-onset growth hormone deficiency were given very low dosages of recombinant human growth hormone or placebo at random for a six-month period. The patients were assessed by using the self-rating Kellner Symptom Questionnaire and the Hamilton Depression Scale. There was no difference in overall scores on the KSQ on entry of the study between the GH and placebo group, nor was there a difference after six months. However, on the Hamilton Depression Scale, the GH group had a decreased score and this correlated directly with increased IGF-1 levels.

There is no reason to settle into a decreased quality of life. With the aid of growth hormone we don't have to consider the apathetic and sedentary lifestyle that comes with age as acceptable. There's no room for the couch potato in us with the supplementation of growth hormone. It's the stimulus of activity and creativity. We've watched our parents and grandparents buckle over with the years. In more unfortunate cases, we've seen our parents or grandparents under attack by age-related diseases like cancer, osteoporosis, heart disease, or mind-altering illnesses like Alzheimer's or Parkinson's disease. The examples our parents have set for us should be the spur to find other methods of aging rather than just giving up the ghost.

Looking Fit and Fabulous

Imagine yourself now that aging has taken an interest in your physical appearance and you're no longer the spring chicken you once were. I'm sure you've noticed your skin isn't as elastic, your belly has gotten bigger, and you're more winded doing menial, daily tasks—like getting the mail, going up the stairs, or keeping up with your children or grandchildren. Your age-related complaints are met with age-related excuses or justifications, and you become accustomed to your new "lifestyle." This doesn't have to be the case. You've read how the supplementation of the other hormones can be the stepping stones to a restored youth as we age; so is the case with growth hormone. It is part of the promise that all the hormones synergistically work together to create—a new, healthier definition of aging.

The physical benefits reported in the 1990 *New England Journal of Medicine* study definitely raised eyebrows of many researchers and doctors interested in the field of longevity medicine. Scientists and doctors already knew that estrogen and testosterone enhanced body shape by decreasing fatty tissue and increasing lean body mass, but the quick results seen in human growth hormone were astounding. Many studies after 1990 have also revealed that, with proper administration of human growth hormone, the visceral fat that accumulates over the years can be reversed within the first six months to a year, in both men and women. One of my patients, "Grace," aged 58, and once a veritable beauty in her day, came to me with hopes of rejuvenation. As with all my patients, I checked her levels and then prescribed the vital and necessary hormones. While stressing that human growth hormone is an elective hormone, supplementation can benefit in ways the other hormones can't. She opted for the full spectrum of therapy. After several months on growth hormone, along with estrogen, testosterone, and progesterone, she came back for a follow-up appointment. She looked fabulous, a mature version of the beauty she once was. She had lost weight, looked vibrant, and boasted of returned youth and energy. Grace is one of many of my favorite personal patient stories, and I believe it to be important to include these stories in this book, but I also think it's important to back them up with tested data. In the *American Journal of Physiology, Endocrinology and Metabolism*, a recent study verified the same benefits found in Grace's experience above. In a randomized placebo-controlled designed study, in addition to a training program, sixteen healthy women aged 75 years were closely monitored for over twelve weeks. The patients who had added growth hormone to their exercise regimen experienced a doubling of insulin-like growth factor I levels. Along with endurance training, both groups experienced an 18 percent increase in peak oxygen intake, but only the growth hormone group showed a marked increase in muscle citrate synthase activity by 50 percent, as well as an increase in other metabolism markers. Although both groups maintained the weight they had at the beginning of the study, the growth hormone group showed significant, positive changes in body composition—a decrease in fat mass and an increase in lean body mass. More astounding is that a twenty-four-hour calorimetry was performed on four of the subjects demonstrating that the two on growth hormone had higher energy expenditure with increased relative and absolute fat combustion. The addition of HGH to the patients' exercise regimen clearly induced desired effects. The women who were administered growth hormone had an age-reversal in their body composition and exercise ability. They basically experienced a setback in aging.

I've seen personally what growth hormone has done in my own life. You come to a certain point in life when you realize your *oomph* is wearing thin and in the case of a doctor, you can only cover a few patient cases in your practice rather than the ten you were once used to. I felt dulled by age, but with the replacement of all the vital hormones, I felt a new breath of life. I experienced what the patients in the next few studies experienced. I watched as my body underwent a total makeover, and this total body readjustment back to youth, helped me to help others.

Many studies illustrate the same wonderful and exciting results. Whether it be long term studies spanning two to ten years or short term studies of six to twelve months, results have been unanimous—human growth hormone replacement reverses the unappealing aspects many of us have grown accustomed to as normal results of aging. In a two-year study, researchers observed growth hormone replacement in adults with growth hormone deficiency. This longer version of previous studies reiterated that growth hormone replacement at optimal levels would produce the desired effects without the forewarned side effects (water retention, joint soreness, carpal tunnel, and hypertension). The study also stressed that patients differ in their need of growth hormone and levels must be titrated to fit each individual's need. In this particular study, body composition altered within three months of its commencement. Lean body mass increased five percent, total body water also increased by five percent, while body fat decreased ten percent. The waist circumference of the growth hormone patients also experienced a slimming and positive change. All this took place within the first year and seemed to attenuate in the second. Yet, what is important is that the subjects did not undergo any strenuous physical training, nor did they alter their diet. The positive physical benefits were purely derived from the supplementation of HGH.

Studies are demonstrating that HGH may have therapeutic benefits on another pressing issue in the United States. It's hard to believe that as many as one third of all adults in America suffer from obesity, which is approximately 70 million people. Each year, obesity results in 300,000 excess deaths and costs the country over 100 billion dollars. With these kinds of statistics, growth hormone replacement therapy actually sounds cost effective. In one specific study, researchers sought to illustrate how growth hormone and dietary restriction can induce accelerated lipolysis (breakdown of stored fat in the cells) and have an anabolic action in obese subjects. A total of twenty-four people were studied, twenty-two women and two men in a twelve-week randomized, double blind, placebo-controlled trial. The difference between the two groups was staggering. Growth hormone treatment caused a 1.6-fold increase in the fraction of body weight lost as fat and a greater loss of visceral fat than the placebo group. The placebo group, even with their restricted calorie intake, experienced a *loss* in lean body mass and experienced a negative nitrogen balance. The growth hormone group, in contrast, increased in lean body mass and had a positive nitrogen balance. GH patients also experienced an increase in IGF-I secretion, despite their caloric restriction. There was no increase in insulin levels in the GH group, yet free fatty acids were significantly decreased which correlated directly with the visceral fat loss. The results in just twelve weeks suggested a possible therapeutic role in one of the most rampant-growing problems facing America today—obesity.

Human growth hormone supplementation can also reverse other outside appearances of age. Patient testimonials along with several documented studies have shown that supplementation of growth hormone can positively alter the texture of aging skin. I'm sure you've noticed the transformation of your skin over the years. It's thinner, translucent, and has lost its youthful elasticity. You can pinch and pull it but instead of snapping back, it stays raised as if it's still being pinched by invisible fingers. The decline of HGH plays a part in this negative adjustment to your skin's beauty. Studies have shown that skin thickness and total skin collagen are reduced in hypopituitary adults. The Rudman study of healthy elderly men with low IGF-I levels showed that skin thickness increased due to the supplementation of growth hormone. In our later years our body water only makes up forty percent of our body mass, a huge discrepancy from the 90 percent in our babyhood or the 60 percent in our adulthood. This dehydration takes the cushion and moistness from the skin, leaving the dried, wrinkled persona of age. HGH helps retain water, although this new-found fluid in the body can sometimes make the joints ache. The ache will disappear with time and titration of dosage, yet the positive effects to the skin will remain.

Some of my patients have also noticed a change in hair growth and color. Other patients have been able to abandon their reading glasses, while others still have detected an overall body and facelift. These are all fascinating stories that generate interest and tempt the taste buds for the fountain of youth. For some patients, grays are replaced by darker hair, glasses are put aside, and bulky clothes and make-up are thrown out with the trash. Your rejuvenation will be as unique as you are yourself.

These are but a few studies that make up a large accumulation of proof for the use of growth hormone for the remodeling of the human body. All around us is evidence of what the aging process can do to the human body. Our metabolism is never quite what it used to be, but now we have the answers—restoration of hormones to their optimal levels can lead us to a restoration of vigor and a youthful appearance. Yet, it's not just the outside appearance that reaps the benefits of growth hormone replacement. HGH also works to ensure health within the body as well. In the next segments, you will learn of growth hormone's far reaching benefits inside our bones as well as some of our vital organs.

HGH: Eliminating the Bone of Contention

As far as human growth hormone is concerned, what is good for the body is good for the bone. The frailty that comes with the adding on of years is not only seen in the wasting away of muscle but bone also suffers an age-related devastation. Our skeletal structure suffers a tremendous amount of remodeling over the years, and as you have learned in earlier chapters, this reworking in not always balanced out or to our benefit. Our bones are torn down faster than they have time to rebuild. Yet, science has found that the addition of natural hormones equalizes bone reconstruction, maintaining a healthy bone mineral density over the years.

This is important since the incidence of osteoporosis is climbing with the growth of the aging population. Medications have been created to treat its symptoms and make them more bearable. Yet, with the information from this book, you can begin to look at osteoporosis and other age-related diseases as illnesses to prevent rather than just treat. This kind of therapy puts a new spin on the kind of medical care that humans have come to accept—wait for the ailment to arise then treat it. As a doctor of longevity medicine, this kind of bide-your-time, doomed medicine defeats the purpose I strive for—treating aging so I won't have to treat the side effects of aging. If we could begin modulating bone density from the get-go, then perhaps such deleterious diseases as osteoporosis or osteoarthritis could be wiped out like smallpox. I believe the supplementation of natural hormones, like human growth hormone, will be a monumental step toward this ultimate goal.

I'm sure you've noticed the common theme threaded throughout this book. With the decline of our essential hormones, necessary activities, like exercise, become much more difficult. I cannot emphasize enough, the differences between a person on natural hormone therapy as compared to a person going without it. One of my hormone therapy patients introduced me to her sister. Although her sister was five years younger, she actually looked ten years older. She lacked the youthful quality—an identifiable lightness in step and clearness of complexion, which hormone replacement can help capture. It truly is a night and day contrast.

In growth hormone deficient patients there is some evidence that bone mass is reduced significantly. This factor suggests that GHD patients have a higher likelihood of suffering from fractures and clinical osteoporosis. Studies have affirmed this theory, although human growth hormone replacement in the realm of osteoporosis therapy is fresh and remains in the study phase. Nonetheless, the results are promising.

A large-scale pharmacoepidemiological survey of adults with

growth hormone deficiency, KIMS (Pharmacia International Metabolic Database) demonstrated a 2.7 times increase of fracture rates over those seen in the control population. Fracture and bone mineral density data from 2024 patients in the KIMS group as compared to the data from 392 patients from the control group illustrated the above increase and showed that its prevalence was more marked in the adult onset, rather than the childhood onset, of the disease. Interestingly enough, the risk of fracture was solely related to growth hormone deficiency rather than other pituitary hormone deficiencies, since with their replacement the condition did not alter.

Beyond this study, endocrinologists, orthopedists, and biophysicists from around the world discussed the advantages and disadvantages on bone density from GH therapy in a 1999 meeting held in Italy. The delegates agreed that it had beneficial effects on bone in adults with growth hormone deficiency and could play an integral role in regulating the fracture rate seen in the elderly all over the world.

Since we're all subject to a decrease of human growth hormone, and some of us are more susceptible to osteoporosis, reason would state that growth hormone replacement, along with enhancing body composition, may also help to enhance skeletal structure. A study of 32 men with adult onset growth hormone deficiency were either given an 18 month trial of growth hormone or a placebo. The study measured both body composition and bone mineral density. The researchers observed that growth hormone had a wonderful influence over bone density of the lumbar spine, increasing it around 5 percent, and the femoral neck, increasing it about 2 percent. The growth hormone group also experienced a healthy bone turnover, seen in the following markers: osteocalcin, urinary puridinoline, and deoxypyridinolone. In a similar fashion, growth hormone swayed body mass—lean body mass increased while adipose tissue decreased. All these healthy changes were significant compared to minor corresponding changes in the placebo group.

Age is heavy-handed with our fate, but unlike centuries ago, we have the methods to weaken or even deter its related diseases and harsh impact. There is no reason to enter into your second adulthood without the natural defense bio-identical hormones can offer your body. You can't put off the years, but you can arrest the age-related complications and age-related physical alterations that getting older can carry with it. Your bones do not have to become brittle and there is no reason you should live in fear of a fracture. Hormones, like growth hormone, can keep your bones as strong as they were in your youth when second-guessing your body never entered your frame of mind. HGH not only influences body make-up and bone turnover, but a huge amount of clinical data is showing that growth hormone may also be an important agent in the fight against heart disease.

Good News for the Weak of Heart

It's a well-known fact, that heart disease is America's number one foe. It's also well known that heart disease rears its head usually after we've hit the fifty-year-mark when many of our life-essential hormones have declined. As I've explained in the preceding chapters, each hormone is helpful to the heart, yet growth hormone has proved to be great news to an already ailing heart. Clinical studies have shown that administration of growth hormone, short term and long term, improves the structural and functional aspects of the heart. Clinical paper after paper and abstract after abstract raises questions on whether or not growth hormone should be in the arena of heart therapy. These questions seem to be answered with proof beyond a doubt that, yes, growth hormone has a place as a therapeutic agent against heart failure. Its applications for the heart are boundless.

I would like to begin this segment with a wonderful story, although, not one of my own, which was reported in a 1999 medical journal. A 63-year-old man with refractory congestive heart failure waiting for a heart transplant and depending on intravenous drugs, was given growth hormone as a last alternative (the unfortunate signature use of growth hormone—as the last alternative). After he was given 8 units per day, doctors noticed a startling improvement. He experienced better optimization of heart failure treatment and was able to discontinue the intravenous drugs. Left ventricular ejection fraction increased from 13 percent to 18 percent, and later to 28 percent with a reduction of pulmonary pressures and an increase in exercise capacity. The patient had such an incredible response to the growth hormone treatment that he was de-listed for heart transplantation.

Of course this could be looked at as some obscure study from some obscure journal, and yes, one man's results cannot determine widespread use of growth hormone for heart patients around the world. Yet, this one study is only an example of what doctors and scientists worldwide are uncovering about growth hormone in regards to an ailing heart. A large database of evidence is compiling year after year that support growth hormone's ability to mend a broken heart. Although the conclusions of these studies stress tentative optimism, its clear heart-healthy benefits can be reaped from its supplementation.

People who suffer from hypopituitarism, and therefore growth hormone deficiency, demonstrate higher risks for cardiac disease. A study in *Lancet* took a retrospective look at patients diagnosed with hypopituitarism between the years1956 through 1987. These patients exhibited an overall elevated chance for mortality, and in regards to vascular disorders, deaths were higher than expected—60 (40 men and 20 women) compared to the 30 that were anticipated. The truth is, patients with advanced clinical manifestations of abnormal GH levels almost always exhibit impaired cardiac function, which may, in fact, reduce life expectancy. These types of studies are important, because whether or not you have a known heart complication, growth hormone, along with other hormones can deter its age-related possibility. Any information toward the possibility of a healthy heart into our eighties and nineties is worthy of taking note of and taking a part in.

The problem is everyone is subject to a decline in growth hormone. At the age of twenty-one, a healthy human body has a normal circulating HGH of ten milligrams per deciliter of blood. At sixty years of age, only about two milligrams per deciliter can be found; the problem being, of course, many doctors look at the two milligrams as being "normal" for an aged adult. You have to be almost bone-dry of HGH to basically get any attention from a health care practitioner. I believe that, as with all hormones, to get optimal results, one should replenish HGH to *optimal* levels—not just to the levels "normal" for their age. Unfortunately, what many doctors look at as "normal" or "sufficient" ranges could lead to impaired glucose tolerance; increased insulin resistance; elevation of serum cholesterol; as well as low-density lipoprotein cholesterol, and decreased high-density lipoprotein. Replacement of the vital hormones, including growth hormone, to our aging bodies can improve the above symptoms of aging and replenish our bodies with the vitality we thought was long gone with our youth.

Plasma lipid profiles are sure indications of heart health. Since many times growth-hormone deficient patients are overweight with reduced lean body mass and increased fat mass, it stands to reason these people have a higher chance of heart failure. This reasoning is confirmed with the common GHD altered substrate metabolism and an abnormal lipid profile. Studies have shown that growth hormone deficient patients have a reduced catabolism (breakdown) of VLDL apoB (the very-low-density lipoprotein or the greatest contributor to atherosclerotic plaque) as compared with control subjects. This slowed metabolic clearance rate indicates that optimal levels of growth hormone are integrally involved in the regulation of VLDL apoB metabolism. This high concentration of VLDL along with low levels of HDL seen in growth hormone deficient patients predisposes them to atherosclerosis and coronary artery disease. Researchers have also uncovered that patients who suffer from a lack of growth hormone show abnormalities in structure and function of the left ventricle along with a significant increase in the vascular intima-media thickness and an increased number of atheromatous plaques—which all boils down to the lack of growth hormone, equaling a greater chance of strokes and heart attacks.

It's well established that growth hormone and IGF-I are modulators of myocardial structure and function. It is also well known that these two components (GH and IGF-I) of the human body are intricately involved in several physiological processes like the control of muscle mass and function, body composition, and regulation of nutrient metabolism. Knowing this and knowing that heart failure is caused by ventricular dilation with abnormal wall thickening, leading to impaired cardiac performance—common sense indicates that growth hormone therapy could curb this event. Many clinical studies point toward this same common sense conclusion.

Several rat models have been used to show the possible use of growth hormone in humans with the predisposition for heart failure. In a particular example, researchers have observed modest increases in cardiac index and stroke volume, coupled with a decrease in systemic vascular resistance, as compared with controls. After fifteen days of growth hormone, the rats also demonstrated reduced left ventricular end-diastolic pressure by 38 percent, indicating a reduction in left-ventricular wall stress. (The left ventricle's importance lies in the fact that it supplies the circulatory system all its blood.) Another study, in regard to left ventricular remodeling, confirmed that rats who had the addition of growth hormone for three weeks displayed a decrease in left ventricular diastolic diameter and an increase in relative wall thickness, along with improvements in cardiac output, stroke volume, and systemic vascular resistance.

Of course, animal studies can only suggest what could happen in human models. Many human studies have replicated the same heart-rejuvenating effects seen in the studies above. One study in particular, cited in the *New England Journal of Medicine*, observed seven patients with idiopathic dilated cardiomyopathy at base line, after three months of therapy with human growth hormone, and three months after the discontinuation of growth hormone. In just three months of therapy researchers discerned that the growth hormone increased left ventricular wall thickness and reduced chamber size significantly. End-systolic wall stress fell markedly while cardiac output was improved, particularly during exercise. The growth hormone improved clinical symptoms: exercise capacity and the patients' quality of life. With the discontinuation of growth hormone, the positive benefits were partially reversed.

Another study, along the same lines, also showed major improvements in hemodynamics and clinical function. Reported in *Circulation*, the journal of the American Heart Association, seven male patients with chronic heart failure due to ischemic heart disease were again studied at baseline, after three months of growth hormone added to the preexisting, conventional therapy, and three months after therapy. The three-month phase of therapy was completed without any adverse side effects. The side benefits were nothing short of amazing. They improved clinically, as indicated by a decreased NYHA (New York Heart Association) functional class. This benefit rapidly decreased after treatment stopped. The patients also demonstrated improvement in exercise capacity (maximal oxygen uptake rose significantly) and the duration of exercise increased dramatically, without a significant alteration of heart rate at rest or during exercise. MRIs showed a significant reduction in end-systolic and end-diastolic volume indexes and an increase in posterior wall thickness, although there was no noteworthy change in left ventricular ejection fraction. Again, some of the positive effects diminished with the discontinuation of growth hormone therapy.

All the above studies may lead you to think that growth hormone is the ultimate elixir for the heart. In some cases it is not. I feel it's my responsibility, as a physician, to have you understand that each patient's affliction is as different as the patient who walks into the doctor's office. One therapy does not work for all, and although it's obvious that growth hormone deficiency causes heart problems, it's also clear, growth hormone in excess (a disease called acromegaly) can have severe effects on the heart as well. Finding the correct balance is of extreme importance. Doctors who use growth hormone therapy should titrate the doses to fit their patients' needs. If you have heart complications, always let your health practitioner know before they start you on *any* regimen. Hormone replacement is not the exception to the rule.

HGH and the Wasting Syndrome

I'm putting this near the end of the chapter, not because it lacks importance, but because it doesn't apply to everyone nor does it always apply to aging. Diseases, like acquired immune deficiency syndrome, have a knack of eating away at their victims. This wasting is defined when a patient involuntarily loses 10 percent of baseline body weight in combination with diarrhea, weakness, or fever. This kind of illness involves a disproportionate loss of lean body mass and muscle wasting. As I've discussed before, and as Rudman famously proved, muscle wasting and poor body composition can be altered with the supplementation of growth hormone—the same kind of results can be seen in patients suffering the deleterious effects of AIDS. The administration of growth hormone has been shown to increase lean body mass and protein synthesis and reduces urinary nitrogen excretion in patients with AIDS and other critical illnesses.

The effects of AIDS on the body can be described as nothing

short of horrific. When a researcher stumbles upon something that can turn around some of the side effects of AIDS, that scientist has found something truly awe-inspiring. Proof of this is shown in a randomized, placebo-controlled study performed in 1996 that showed how the supplementation of growth hormone to 178 patients with AIDS wasting had body- and health-altering positive benefits. The treated patients gained lean body mass and weight, yet lost fat and also had an increase in total body and intracellular water. These patients also showed vast improvements of exercise ability as seen in treadmill performance. Therefore, their quality of life experienced an unexpected boost.

In the case of critical illnesses, like AIDS, human growth hormone is a genuine healer. Although it is in no way a cure, its persuasion over body composition and energy levels are reason enough to take notice. Growth hormone has the power to restore youth to an aging body and mind and restore a strong semblance of health in an ailing body. This hormone has amazing and far-reaching benefits that should not be ignored or bogged down by the orthodox medical community.

One example of this kind of biased, conservative medicine is seen in the study by Takala et al. that declared growth hormone, administered to severely ill patients, increased mortality rather than prolonging it. He showed a 42 percent increase of mortality, which superceded the 18 percent increase in the placebo group. These statistics, of course are frightening. Before you decide against growth hormone, you should take into consideration that the high doses these patients were administered were unconventional and not modified per patient need. Second of all, other scientists in light of these kind of tragic results have analyzed the KIMS database, the Pharmacia and Upjohn International Metabolic DATABASE, (the largest database of patients on growth hormone therapy) to assess whether Takala's results are valid. What they found is gratifying for me as a doctor who prescribes growth hormone and of course for my patients that use it. The KIMS database showed that growth hormone replacement was <u>not</u> associated with increased mortality. They also emphasized that the dosage used in Takala's study was *ten times* that which was used in the KIMS analysis. Ten times the amount in drug therapy can truly make the difference and in the case of mortality, it was an irresponsible step in the wrong direction.

It's always important to cover all your bases when someone makes a rather bold statement as Takala and his group did. When searching out answers and the perfect therapy for you, it's good to do your own meta-analysis. With the clinical studies that I have littered throughout this chapter, you can see that growth hormone's benefits, if properly dosed, supercede any negative feedback you may have heard regarding its supplementation.

Why I Propose a Name Change for Human Growth Hormone

The name human growth hormone sometimes confuses people. They see the word "growth" and they negatively associate it with cancer. Growth hormone does not cause or spur cancer, dormant or malignant, to grow. HGH is only called growth hormone because it is the main hormone responsible for linear growth in our puberty years. Its lack, therefore, is the direct cause of dwarfism. To clear up the confusion, I believe HGH should be renamed the "Human Healing Hormone" due to its dramatic effects on healing the body against disease and injury.

The *New England Journal of Medicine* performed a world or meta-analysis on literature pertaining to growth hormone, and instead of finding an increase in cancer from the use of growth hormone, they found a 50 percent decrease in the risk of cancer. Unfortunately, many physicians are not aware of this study. Many times doctors criticize not because they understand but rather from lack of experience or knowledge of the tremendous benefits of growth hormone. I believe it's a kind of survival technique—doctors ignore or disparage what they don't know, so they never have to admit ignorance. I use this article weekly to argue the case of human growth hormone supplementation with doctors across the board. There is too much riding on a fate without it—and I don't know about you, but I'm not about to settle into an increase of visceral fat, decreased mobility, and a heightened risk of heart disease. This fairy tale that HGH causes cancer or instigates cancer is just that, a fairy tale, proven in the *New England Journal of Medicine.*

As with all hormones, there may be transitory, minor side effects with commencement. With growth hormone the side effects are edema (swelling of the joints), joint pain or stiffness, or carpel tunnel syndrome—cancer is not one of them. These inconveniences can be eliminated with proper administration and dosing by an experienced practitioner. The best tool of the trade is to start low and go slow. It's best to start at a low dosage and slowly raise it. This will help to eliminate the chance of side effects.

Make sure you understand your own motivations. Beginning a replacement program should be a lifelong pursuit and commitment. After you've restored your hormones to optimal levels, and experience the liveliness they evoke, you will not want to return to the baseline levels you were at when you started. Once you stop, you won't experience a rough transition, nor will your body suffer complications of producing hormones on its own; your levels will merely drop to where they were before. In this way, aging is now a matter of *choice*.

How to Recognize a Scam When You See It

There have been instances when several of my patients have called to let me know they have found a source of HGH much cheaper than what they have been getting through a pharmacy. It's true you can find a fountain of alleged "human growth hormone" supplements over the Internet. But watch out. These companies are very sly and deceptive about how they market their oral or transdermal products. They cite actual recombinant growth hormone studies, refer potential customers to books on HGH, and employ testimonials for that final, hard sale. This kind of advertising is irresponsible and entirely false. Such sites unabashedly make claims that their products produce the same effects as HGH and many times go above and beyond touting benefits that even real human growth hormone cannot offer. Here are just a few examples of the kind of extremities these manufacturers will go to:

> *I would say this product took a good ten years off the look of my face. My skin is tighter, smoother, firmer and has a youthful glow.*

This next testimonial is after just one month of use:

> ...my sister who is diabetic and could hardly get out bed till noon is now jumping up everyday at sunrise like I have never seen her before....My pants are falling off from the fat I have lost and muscle tone has definitely increased.

And this example makes me laugh to myself every time:

> Fact: Sprays are an ineffective fad because human growth hormone is a large, unstable molecule that can't pass through membranes in the mouth. They contain potentially dangerous binders and fillers, additives which must be avoided. Our formula is a liquid tincture and the only one using the powerful Alpha Trisequelene for delivery.

The above statement is very misleading in that it uses the tactic of truth. Sprays *are* ineffective because of the large molecular size of HGH, yet they failed to admit that HGH in liquid form, whether it be alcohol based or not, cannot boost HGH levels either. And that big word they used, smack dab in the middle of it, means nothing but a smart marketing ploy. All you'll learn about how this "patented trade secret" is an amazing miracle, yet, you'll never see any studies verifying its purpose and potency. These sites are full of half-lies with half-truths and distinguishing between the two can get pretty ridiculous for a public unaware of the differences between actual recombinant growth hormone and a growth hormone "stimulator." This chapter, in part, is to educate you on the wonderful benefits of growth hormone supplementation. The other part is to warn you against the products that arouse great expectations, yet deliver little reward.

These products are supposedly endorsed by sports stars and "M.D.'s" One site in particular used a quote from a Harvard trained neurosurgeon, stressing, of course, the source of his education. I would like to emphasize that the initials M.D. do not always mean that the information is truthful. Doctors, whether they have graduated from Harvard or not, are not always honest about the products in question, and many times you'll find these doctors have a monetary motive to endorse a product, rather than a clinical incentive. Unless they have hard data or information you can check elsewhere, beyond just their website and promotional material, you should steer clear from products promising the effects of human growth hormone without actually *being* human growth hormone. If they do claim to have growth hormone, it's a minuscule amount, being over-the-counter, and is null nonetheless because its molecular size makes it impossible, in its mode of administration, to be absorbed across the cell membrane.

As of yet, the only way human growth hormone can be supplemented is if it's administered through an injection. Its molecular structure is too large that any other way is impossible to absorb. Human growth hormone is made up of 191 amino acids, making it longer than insulin, which as you well know has to also be injected. Its molecular size makes it impossible to traverse the membrane structure of the intestine and therefore, the protease in the stomach breaks it down into separate amino acids. Alone these amino acids may have positive influences on the body, but by no means do they have the effect of growth hormone. Powders, creams, pills or drops are, therefore, not HGH, and most likely you will be wasting your money and energy in their purchase. The only benefit these products can evoke is by way of boosting the natural secretion of growth hormone by influencing your pituitary gland. Even then, this is usually only seen in younger patients, not in the older, sedentary patients that are truly in need of it. In truth, you can get the same burst of growth hormone secretion from lifting weights as you can get from taking a HGH booster. So, I advise you to save your money for the benefits of the real growth hormone.

Secretagogues, and the like, have left a sour taste in my mouth for more than the reason that they don't work. It's the kind of dishonesty the manufacturers use to tantalize the hopeful, that bothers me. Like most products out there, be skeptical and check their sources, just as I encourage you to check mine. Your health is at stake and you should be aware of what and why you put something in your body.

Where Do I Go For Rejuvenation?

Rejuvenation is not just a human growth hormone responsibility. Although you'll read from other sources that it's the panacea of the century, I believe that alone it can only do so much. Optimal rejuvenation is achieved through a combination of *all* the vital hormones. Women who seek strong bones need the bone healthy supplementation of natural estrogen and testosterone. If they seek an elixir for the heart and mind, natural estrogen and progesterone should be added to their medicinal regimen. If men desire a youthful figure and an energy boost, a stronger heart and resilient bones, they should seek out a source for supplemental testosterone and DHEA. Human growth hormone is an enhancer to the above hormone-supplemented benefits. Some believe it goes above and beyond what the other hormones can do, and yes, in a way it does. Its effects are fast acting (example seen in the Rudman study)—yet, for optimal health, for a youthful sex drive, for endless energy, for an emotional boost, and memory enhancement—all hormones must be optimally supplemented.

The search for youth is not always easy. You may run into obstacles from all sides. Your family may think you're crazy and dabbling in hokey medicine. Your general practitioner may find this "hormone quackery" a waste of time and money, and your friends may think it's a sign of a midlife crisis. I consider the term "mid-life crisis" to be right on. Your body is in shock from the lack of the essential hormones, and it's acting accordingly. When I saw myself aging and the zest for my career and for my hobbies waning, I felt like I was in a serious quandary. I began what I call the futile quarrel with my body, which rebelled against my every push. It wasn't until I found the source of healthy aging in natural hormone replacement, that I could stop this fruitless fight against getting older. I ended my midlife crisis, not through destructive methods—like finding myself in a financial predicament of divorce or buying a new and impractically expensive car. Instead, I restored my hormones to the optimal levels they once were in my youth, and I again felt alive and at the wheel. I haven't put time on hold, nor have I suspended the years, but I am healthier and full of energy. I have, in a sense, interrupted the historic idea of growing older, since mine is a healthy and enjoyable aging.

As for your doctor, maybe this would be a good book for him/her to read. If they're worried about overuse, or the hormone has been stigmatized by reports of growth hormone abuse by sports stars, then I suggest he consider opening himself up to other reasons people use HGH. Growth hormone is no different than other hormones in that it is essential for the maintenance of good health and quality of life. Optimizing the levels of growth hormone, as well as the other hormones, can prevent deterioration caused by aging. It is not whether studies back up the claims of rejuvenation, but whether your doctors will open themselves beyond the one-size-fits-all concept of medicine.

Finding someone equipped with the clinical know-how of bio identical hormone replacement is not easy, but there are doctors who do practice this therapy. Make sure you understand their motives and experience. Also seek a doctor concerned about your symptoms and requests, not just about your test results. Look for someone who wants to be a partner in your longevity. Indeed, it is the rest of your life you're planning out—it should be considered with both solemnity and anticipation.

As you head into your future with the desire to improve your quality of life, you may find that you have to go outside the boundaries of our conservative healthcare system. "Preventive medicine" is rarely recognized or endorsed by insurance plans and if hormone replacement is approved, it's approved only for the pharmaceutical industry's synthetic hormones. Only the progressive health plans have added compounding pharmacies to their programs. So, as you journey into a healthier aging, be prepared to pay for your prescriptions out of your own pocket—although, you may be surprised that it's not that expensive and in the scheme of things, preventing disease and age-related complications is more cost-effective than treating a disease.

I implore you to ignore the narrow-minded world of conventional medicine, which considers aging and its pitfalls to be a natural, albeit painful, part of living into your eighties or nineties. Study after study shows that proper supplementation of hormones, like that of growth hormone, can offer you the energy and motivation to make those years some of the most enticing moments of your life. I offer hormone replacement therapy to others because of what it offered me—a future not weighed down by reflecting on and pining for years of a youth now gone. With hormone replacement therapy, I, along with many of my patients, can finally say, "youth is not wasted on the young."

Talking the Talk Your Doctors Understand

Many physicians and patients require proof from our medical literature that optimal hormone replacement is both beneficial and safe. There is a plethora of information and data in peer-reviewed medical journals that frequently goes unrecognized and unappreciated. The following are direct quotes from well-recognized and esteemed medical journals in the world. These journals are widely accepted by authorities to be legitimate and well researched.

The reason I'm including this point-by-point reference on some of the major hormones I've profiled in this book is so that you will have a foundation of data with which to approach your doctor. I think it's important to understand the fundamentals behind the argument for a healthier aging, and this allows you to reference important studies that validate this kind of medicine. I wish you good luck in your quest for knowledge and achievement of a better quality of life and a healthier longevity.

Human Growth Hormone

Geriatrics: November, 1999; vol. 54:11 pg. 62.

- The length between obesity and diseases of aging has been confirmed.

• Increase in visceral fat tissue has a direct effect on age associated insulin resistance and cardiovascular disease. The increase of visceral fat in older persons is associated with the decreased levels of estrogen, testosterone, and growth hormone.
• Augmenting the levels of these and other hormones that decrease with age better controls visceral fat, thereby leading to decreased insulin resistance, decreased diabetes, and decreased atherosclerosis.

New England Journal of Medicine: October, 1999 vol. 341: pgs1206-1216.

• In adults the goals of growth hormone replacement are to restore normal body composition, improve muscle and cardiac function, normalize serum lipid concentrations, and improve quality of life.
• There is evidence that growth hormone deficiency in adults is deleterious, increasing the risk of death from cardiovascular disease.
• There is, at present, no evidence that growth hormone replacement therapy affects the risk of cancer or cardiovascular disease. Studies show the rate of mortality from cancer was either half the rate of normal subjects or similar to it.
• After six months of treatment the basal metabolic rate increased by 6 percent to 11 percent. (This means that the metabolism has increased, which in turn burns body fat.)
• Medical studies show that quality of life measures, including energy level, mood, and emotions, improve with the supplementation of growth hormone. There is a significant improvement of scores in standard psychological tests of energy, emotions, and well-being.
• Changes in metabolic rate and in muscle and fat mass allow patients to become more physically active.

JAMA: August, 2000 vol. 284: 7 pgs 861-866.

• From young adulthood to midlife growth hormone secretion decreases by 75 percent. Somatapause or loss of growth hormone is essentially completed by the fourth decade.

• Data shows that we should target a younger age for replacement therapy, rather than those older than 65, in order to prevent exposure of low growth hormone levels for at least two decades.

Psychoneuroendocrinology: 1992 vol. 17:4 pgs 327-333.

• Growth hormone administration increases muscle mass, improves exercise tolerance, improves REM sleep, and enhances a sense of well-being.

Hospital Medicine: September, 1999 pg. 29.

• Growth hormone replacement significantly increases patients' lean body mass and decreases fat mass.

New England Journal of Medicine: 1990;323: pgs1-6.

• Effects of six months of human growth hormone administration on lean body mass and adipose tissue mass were equivalent in magnitude to the changes incurred during ten-twenty years of aging.

Hormone Research: 1991;35 (1):19-24.

• We conclude that exogenous growth hormone administration reduces body fat in obese women in the apparent absence of significant kilo-caloric restriction.

Clinical Endocrinology: 1992;37: 79-87.

• Growth hormone therapy increased lean body mass and decreased fat mass. The sense of general well-being improved in most patients.

Annals of Internal Medicine: 1996;125(11)889-90.

• Administered growth hormone increases bone density and

stimulates bone turnover, decreases body fat and increases lean body mass, and is associated with a low incidence of side effects.

Schweiz Med Wochenschr: 1997;127 (35):1440-9

- These studies have led to the recognition of a specific syndrome of GH deficiency, characterized by symptoms and signs.
- Adults with long-standing growth hormone deficiency are often overweight, have altered body composition—reduced lean body mass, increased fat mass, reduced total body water and reduced bone mass.
- ...there is a reduced physical and cardiac performance.
- ...there is a reduced psychological well-being and quality of life.
- GH treatment restores lean body mass, reduces fat mass, increases total body water and increases bone mass.
- ...psychological well-being and quality of life improve with replacement therapy.

Journal of Clinical Endocrinology and Metabolism: 1999;84:2596-2602.

- Growth hormone treatment for 10 years in growth hormone deficient adults resulted in increased lean body and muscle mass, a less atherogenic lipid profile, reduced carotid intima media thickness, and improved psychological well-being.

Testosterone

Journal of Clinical Endocrinology and Metabolism: 1996;81:3578-83.

- The author concluded that testosterone replacement in androgen-deficient men improved positive mood parameters, including friendliness, well-being, and energy, while decreasing negative mood.

Archives of Family Medicine: 1999;8:257-263.

- The clinical manifestation of androgen deficiency depends on

the age at onset and severity and duration of the deficiency,
- 	…included reduced body hair, decreased muscle mass and strength, increased fat mass, decreased hematocrit (decreased red-blood cell count), decreased libido, erectile dysfunction, infertility, osteoporosis, and depressed mood.
- 	For most patients, androgen replacement therapy with testosterone is a safe, effective treatment for testosterone deficiency.
- 	The most accurate indicator of hypogonadism is the concentration of testosterone that is not bound to sex-hormone-binding-globulin (the concentration of bio-available testosterone known as free testosterone.)
- 	Benefits of androgen replacement therapy include increased body hair and beard growth, energy, red blood cell count, muscle mass, strength and stamina
- 	…increased ability to perform more physically demanding tasks
- 	…overall increase in the sense of well-being, confidence, and motivation
- 	bone mineral density is increased by testosterone replacement
- 	improved libido and sexual function

Obesity Research: 1995;3:609S

- 	Testosterone therapy was also followed by a specific decrease of visceral fat mass (measured by CT scan), by increased insulin sensitivity (measured with the euglycemic glucose clamp), by decrease in fasting blood glucose, plasma cholesterol, and triglycerides as well as a decrease in diastolic blood pressure.

Diabetes & Metabolism (Paris):1995;21:156-161.

- 	Further work is required to determine whether and why physiologic testosterone levels in the high normal range appear to be conducive to optimal cardiovascular health for adult men.
- 	Adult men with high normal concentrations of endogenous testosterone have more favorable levels of several major heart disease

risk factors, including HDL-cholesterol, a more suitable fat pattern, and lower glucose and insulin levels than do men with low testosterone concentrations.
• Nearly all the observations support the notion that men should be men, hormonally speaking, for the prevention of heart disease.

Proceedings of the National Academy of Science USA: 1997;94:6612-6617.

• Recent reports have identified a protective effect of estrogen in the development of Alzheimer's disease, and new studies show that testosterone may exert an even stronger preventive effect.
• ...testosterone may exert a greater neuroprotective effect than estrogen.

Proceedings of the National Academy of Science of USA: 2000;97:1202-05.

• Alzheimer's disease (AD) is characterized by the age related deposit of beta-amyloid peptide aggregates in vulnerable areas.
• Studies have reported that estrogen replacement therapy protects against the development of AD in postmenopausal women.
• Increasing evidence indicates that testosterone, especially bio-available testosterone, decreases with age in older men and in postmenopausal women.
• ...treatment with testosterone increases the secretion of the nonamyloidogenic APP fragment, spAPP alpha, and decreases the secretion of A beta peptides from nerve cells. The results raise the possibility that testosterone supplementation in elderly men may be protective in the treatment of AD.

Executive Director of the Broda O. Barnes, MD Research Foundation

• Symptoms of male climacteric can include decreased libido or loss of sexual desire, depression, muscle weakness, pain and stiffness, excessive seating with intolerance to heat, irritability, and heart irregularities.

- Too many men who experience these symptoms will suffer in silence and accept them as the inevitable signs of aging.
- Some information that is not commonly known about testosterone is that it is cardiac-protective.
- …is one of the major regulators of fat and protein and sugar metabolism. Testosterone is also effective in the prevention and treatment of bone loss. This information is well-documented in medical literature.
- This form of testosterone (methyl-testosterone) is harmful to the liver….
- ….be sure to ask your physician for the natural testosterone preparation which is readily available.

Urology: 1991;XXXVII, number 3.

- …restoring normal erectile activity with an increased frequency of ejaculation has a positive effect on both mood and energy.
- There was no change in prostate or urinary flow and frequency.
- There were no dermatologic problems associated with the system, the tenfold increase in DHT over baseline levels was attributed to 5-alpha reduction of testosterone in the scrotal skin.
- …the goal of maintaining serum testosterone concentration within the physiologic range.

Journal of Women's Health: 1998;7(7):825-9.

- The ovaries are a critical source not only of estrogen but also of testosterone
- Women who have had a hysterectomy have three times the risk of cardiovascular disease compared with women who have not.
- Restoring a physiologic level of testosterone to women after a hysterectomy not only can improve quality of life in terms of libido, sexual pleasure, and sense of well-being but also can build bones, and may be a key to protecting cardiovascular health.

New England Journal of Medicine: 2000;343:682-8.

- ...the higher testosterone dose resulted in further increases in scores for frequency of sexual activity and pleasure-orgasm in the Brief Index of Sexual Functioning for Women.
- ...the percentages of women who had sexual fantasies, masturbated, or engaged in sexual intercourse at least once a week increased two to three times the baseline.
- The positive well-being, depressed-mood, and composite scores of the Psychological General Well-Being Index also improved at the higher dose.
- ...transdermal testosterone improves sexual function and psychological well-being.
- Finally, transdermal testosterone was not associated with clinically important changes in acne, hirsutism, or laboratory test results.
- Treatment with the higher dose of testosterone improved sexual function and psychological well-being substantially more than placebo treatment.

JAMA: 2000;283: number 20.

- Androgens appear to have an important effect on women's energy and well-being.
- ...particularly in relation to depression. Improvements in libido were also reported.
- Lack of energy is one of the factors that most negatively affect the quality of life for many menopausal and post-menopausal women.
- I would consider treating a woman with a level of free testosterone below the midpoint of the normal range for the available assay.
- The potential for this research is phenomenal.

Thyroid

Annals of Internal Medicine: 2000;132:270-8.

- Subclinical hypothyroidism is linked with a more-than-twofold increase in heart attack risk among women aged 55 and older, according to a recent study from the Netherlands.
- ...mild thyroid disease is in the same ballpark as well-estab-

lished cardiac risk factors like high cholesterol and smoking.
- …it does tip the balance toward recommending thyroid replacement therapy, which is a relatively benign treatment, to your patients who have this common condition.

Mayo Clinic for Women's HealthSource

- You're tired. You have mood swings, sleep problems and your periods are irregular. You notice changes in the texture of your hair and shine and you're often anxious and irritable. Symptoms like these are easy to dismiss or just as easy to blame on aging, stress, monthly hormonal fluctuations, or menopause.
- These symptoms can be a sign that your thyroid is acting up.
- In fact, your overall body functioning is dependent on you thyroid hormones

New England Journal of Medicine: 1999;340:424-9.

- Combined therapy with thyroxine and triiodothyronine may be an improvement over standard thyroxine treatments for patients with hypothyroidism.
- Although generally effective, not all patients benefit from thyroxine treatment
- …the combination therapy group scored their mood as significantly improved
- …physical well-being is significantly better on three of the seven scales. No test scores for patients on thyroxine alone showed any improvement.
- These patients reported having more energy, better concentration, and an improved sense of well-being.

American Journal of Cardiology: 1998;81:443-447.

- Most patients with advanced congestive heart failure have altered thyroid hormone metabolism. A low triiodothyronine level is associated with impaired hemodynamics and is an independent predictor of poor survival.

Journal of Gerontology: Medical Sciences 1999;54A(3):M111-M116.

• Our data suggests that older subjects may require circulating thyroid hormones in middle to high levels in order to maintain optimal brain functioning.
• ...variations in these levels can have significant cognitive consequences, even apparently in euthyroid subjects.
• Therefore, it is quite possible that there is a substantial population of undetected, subclinically hypothyroid individuals in the general population who may suffer subtle cognitive deficits, long before hypothyroidism manifests by obvious metabolic symptoms. Although thyroid supplementation of subclinical patients has been relatively uncommon, it is gaining support.

Annals of Internal Medicine: 2000;132:270-278.

• Hypothyroidism is accompanied by a hypercoagulable state, increased blood viscosity, and a greater plasma concentration of homocysteine.
• Subclinical hypothyroidism is a strong indicator of risk of atherosclerosis and myocardial infarction in elderly women.

Estrogen

Geriatrics: 1996;51(8):16.

• Women are skeptical about estrogen replacement therapy. They are unconvinced about its efficacy. Side effects are reported as the primary reason for discontinuing therapy. Physicians and patients require continuing education to emphasize estrogen's potential benefits.

Biomedicina: 2000;3(1):5-20.

• Estrogen improves quality of life, decreases hot flashes, night sweats, and depression. Estrogen maintains youthful appearance,

avoids wrinkles, improves sex-life. Estrogen keeps strong and healthy bones from deteriorating. Estrogen avoids heart problems, memory loss.
- Estrogen enhances skin smoothness, firmness, and elasticity. Estrogen moistens skin and mucus membranes and prevents urogenital atrophy. Estrogen prevents sexual dysfunction.
- Estrogen reduces the risk of heart disease, osteoporosis, colon cancer, improves memory and neurologic function, prevents against Alzheimer's disease, enhances immune function, and improves well-being.
- Estrogen preserves independence, prevents morbidity, and enhances well-being.

Hospital Practice: August, 1999: 102.

- Estrogen dramatically reduces the risk of cardiovascular disease in women by up to 50 percent. This effect was felt to be through improvement of the lipid profile.
- Most of the survival benefit has been found to stem from a direct antiatherosclerotic, anticoagulatory, and vasodilatary effects of estrogen. (The recent HERS study showed an increased risk of heart attack in women taking estrogen if they had a prior history of cardiovascular disease. This is a very small percentage of women, overall. It is due to congenital clotting abnormalities and is an extremely small percent of the total population. Most healthy women will benefit from this replacement.)
- Estrogen therapy has been shown to significantly reduce the risk of macular degeneration by 70 percent. (Currently this is the only proven therapy to slow down the most common cause of blindness in our society.)
- Superior dental health of estrogen users was the result of bone preservation and maintenance of collagen in the supporting gingival structures.
- Estrogen reduces the incidence of urogenital complaints such as vaginal dryness, urinary infection, and loss of supporting structures. (This should give women something to smile about.)

Infertility and Reproductive Medicine Clinics of North America: October, 1995;6(4):653-660.

•   This manuscript presents a protocol for hormone replacement therapy using
    natural estrogen, testosterone, DHEA, and progesterone.
•   Serum hormone levels are measured and replaced to premenopausal levels using the natural hormones. We believe this method of hormone replacement therapy is based on sound physiological principles. It ensures establishment of premenopausal levels of circulating sex steroids. (This was a landmark article in the obstetric/gynecology literature that went unnoticed. This excellent article not only discusses the method of replacement, but also emphasizes the lack of side effects associated with this therapy as it maintains premenopausal levels of the natural hormones as opposed to using the synthetic, which were associated with a significantly higher incidence of side effects. Remember as stated at the beginning, women stop estrogen therapy because of side effects. Using natural hormones eliminates these side effects and significantly increases compliance.)

Archives of Dermatology: 1997;133: 339-342.

•   Estrogen therapy is associated with a significant decrease in skin wrinkling and skin dryness in women, increase in dermal and total skin thickness, and preservation of skin texture.
•   There is a 30 percent decrease of collagen after menopause, resulting in loss of skin thickness and elasticity. These changes are reversible with estrogen replacement therapy. (If that will not increase compliance, I don't know what will.)

Consultant Magazine: December, 2000: 2312.

•   Multiple epidemiologic and observational studies from more than 27 studies performed over the last two decades demonstrate a significant reduction in heart disease mortality in women who took hormone therapy.

Chemical Research and Toxicology: 1999;12(2):204-13.

•   A major metabolite of equilin auto-oxidized to a potent uncogenic metabolite equilenin, a component of Premarin is easily metabolized to cytotoxic metabolites that can stimulate breast tumors. (Natural hormones follow normal metabolic pathways so that the active metabolites formed are easily metabolized by the body. Therefore, administration of bio-identical hormones to humans can eliminate the production of problem causing metabolites, which are probably responsible for the side effects as well as the increased cancer incidence of the synthetic hormones.)

Obstetrics and Gynecology: 1989;73:606.

•   Women that were prescribed natural estrogen and natural progesterone had a decrease in total cholesterol and an increase of HDL. Those on synthetic conjugated estrogens and medroxyprogesterone (Provera) had no change. This study demonstrates that administration of natural hormones results in symptomatic improvement, minimal side effects, improved lipid profile, and protection of the uterus. (Again another article from our medical literature supporting the use of natural hormones to avoid side effects and complications of the synthetics.)

Progesterone

American Family Physicians: 2000;62(8):1839.

•   The multitude of side effects associated with the synthetic analogues called progestins has stimulated an interest in natural progesterone. Natural progesterone is obtained primarily from plant sources. Natural progesterone has improved bioavailability and fewer side effects when compared with synthetic progestins.

•   Natural progesterone has not been shown to effect mood or cholesterol levels. The synthetic progestins differ from the natural progesterone since they cause fluid retention, abnormal increase in cholesterol, headaches, mood disturbance, depression, and are frequently a cause of discontinuation of hormone therapy. (Again adequate documentation in our literature of the protective benefits of natural progesterone without all the side effects of synthetics. It is very well supported in our medical literature, yet unfortunately unrecognized by most physicians.)

Mayo Clinic, Women's HealthSource: August, 1999, pg 3.

•   Women prefer the use of natural progesterone over synthetic progestins. Natural progesterone made a difference in overall quality of life, menopausal symptoms, and satisfaction.
•   Natural progesterone is not associated with the abnormal metabolites from synthetic progestins. These abnormal metabolites are substances that are responsible for the side effects. Natural progesterone is the same substance you are making naturally, and therefore side effects are avoided.

American Family Physician: 1999;16(1):264.

•   Synthetic progestins produce undesirable side effects, making natural progesterone a better alternative. The side effects of the synthetics, including bloating, nausea, and depression, were eliminated by using natural progesterone. In fact, unexpected improvement in the feeling of well-being was observed when natural progesterone was used.

Journal of Women's Health Gender-based Medicine: 2000;9(4):381-7.

•   When compared to the synthetic progestins, women using micronized, natural progesterone experienced significant improvement in symptoms without the side effects of the synthetics. The natural progesterone offers improvement in quality of life in comparison with the synthetic progestin.

DHEA

Journal of Clinical Endocrinology and Metabolism: June,

1994;78(6):1360-7.

- ...serum levels were restored to those found in young adults within 2 weeks of DHEA replacement.
- ...increase in serum levels of androgens (androstenedione, testosterone, and dehydrotestosterone) was observed in women.
- ...small rise in androstenedione in men.
- ...serum IGF-I levels increased significantly.
- ...associated with a remarkable increase in perceived physical and psychological well-being for both men (67%) and women (84%)
- These observations together with improvement of physical and psychological well-being in both genders and the absence of side effects constitute the first demonstration of novel effects of DHEA replacement in age-related symptoms of both men and women.

Journal of Clinical Investment: August, 1998;82(2):712-20.

- DHEA is an endogenous steroid that blocks carcinogenensis, retards aging, and exerts antiproliferative properties.
- ...low levels of DHEA or its sulfate conjugate are linked to an increase risk of developing cancer or of death from cardiovascular disease.
- The results show that high levels of plasma DHEA inhibit the development of atherosclerosis and they provide an important experimented link to the epidemiologic studies correlating low DHEA-sulfate plasma levels with an enhanced risk of cardiovascular mortality.

Annals of NY Academy of Sciences: December, 1995;774:271-80.

- This data suggests that low plasma levels of DHEA may facilitate, and high levels may retard, the development of coronary atherosclerosis and coronary allograft vasculopathy.

World Congress on Osteoporosis

- After one year, bone mineral density differed significantly between DHEA-treated and placebo-treated women at several sites.

• In general, BMD increased in those treated with DHEA and decreased in those who took placebo.
• Serum telopeptide of type 1 collagen, an indicator of bone resorption, decreased by 11 percent after 6 months and by 26 percent after 1 year.

American Journal of Physiology: November, 1997;273(5 pt 2):R1704-8.
• Results show that DHEA has a protective effect against accumulation of visceral fat and development of muscle, and insulin resistance in rats fed a high-fat diet.

Epilogue:
Making the Choice for a Healthy Longevity

Just a couple of days ago I received a postcard from two of my patients, a husband and wife vacationing in the Caribbean for a month. They wrote: "Enjoying the sun, enjoying each other, enjoying our seventies. Thanks." A simple statement, really, but packed with so much meaning. This is what is important to understand if nothing else as you read this book—through natural hormone replacement therapy, you can truly begin to understand what it's like to enjoy life for the rest of your life; whether you are forty-five or seventy-nine or eighty-six, it's never too late to discover a healthier aging.

USA Today Snapshots features contemporary trivia about how we as a nation feel about our healthcare and culture. In a current "snapshot" *USA Today* tallied the biggest concerns Americans have about growing older. The number one fear, 83%, was the "slowing down" side effect associated with aging. Following closely, at 81%, was an unease regarding "overall health," and at 56%, many people worried about becoming a "family burden." I started this book with why I began the journey into a healthier aging. I, like many Americans, saw that my own downward spiral was imminent. I felt the first stings of aging at forty-three and I too agonized over slowing down, a flagging health, and becoming a burden to my wife (although, I'm sure there are times she already sees me as one). This concern for my health spurred me to become my own guinea pig in an experiment, which I hoped would reap a more fruitful future. Lucky for me, it did. Yet, I realized that my own experiences could not be reason enough for me to feel secure in prescribing hormones to my patients (although, in truth, I wanted to share how good I felt with whole world). Instead, I delved into medical texts and journals, stockpiled studies past and present, and kept my ears and eyes open for any new developments on the horizon. What I found was monumental proof—our quality of life, our health and happiness dwindle seemingly at the same rate our hormone levels decrease and with their restoration our bodies and minds can again enjoy the health and vigor allotted by youth. This conclusion is apparent in the many studies that spice the chapters of this book—our hormones keep us healthy and when restored to optimal ranges, they keep us energetic and youthful. This was reason enough to devote my attention and medical know-how to my patients' healthy longevity.

Where We Stand Today

We live on the cusp of a new science and medicine, a field that I, along with a minority of doctors, have been working in long before it became as popular as it is today. The baby boomers and their offspring are a lucky group of people, in that they live in a world of changing perceptions about aging and its associated harbingers of deterioration and illness. Undeniably, you will still encounter the habitual outlook on aging as something unavoidable and more often than not unendurable, yet I'm sure you're becoming familiar with a new attitude, as you watch TV and read popular magazines like *Time* or *Newsweek*, that aging and its related complexities are being transformed from a normal way of aging to something that can be avoided by healthy living and supplementation of natural hormones and vitamins and minerals. I wrote this particular book to substantiate many of those claims the popular media is making, with hardcore evidence from prestigious medical journals and from my own experiences as a doctor in the field of natural, bio identical hormone replacement therapy. With this book, I wanted to open you to that possibility of aging without really aging, and that opportunity to enjoy your fifties, sixties, seventies, etc. with the same energy and passion you enjoyed during your twenties and thirties.

Yet, although there is ample clinical data compiled in this book and elsewhere regarding the benefits of natural hormone replacement, there is a prevalence in our mainstream culture of a fear, instigated more out of ignorance of this new strain of medicine, than out of genuine insight. Therefore, I would like to, as I conclude this book, venture a rebuttal to the negative news about the whole spectrum of longevity medicine. As you read the newspaper and popular magazines I can assure you that you will find arguments forming about whether this kind of program is right for you. A perfect example of this was demonstrated just recently, in the September 2001 *Newsweek*. This issue was devoted entirely to the question of "Living Longer and Living Better." The articles were well written, some of them rather engaging; yet, I was appalled at the lack of scientific responsibility in some of their statements, specifically about hormone replacement. My first warning to you as a well-educated and curious reader is that articles concerning hormone replacement are usually centered on the chemically-altered hormones, like Provera or Premarin. You cannot imply that the outcomes of hormones, molecularly altered, will be the same as outcomes from the use of natural hormones—created to fit human receptor sites like a lock and key mechanism. Your hormones have kept you healthy thus far, and deductive reasoning supports that supplementing with the exact replica would result in the same healthy effect. I also ask you to be wary of one-sided coverage, and in this case, especially note who funded the entire September 2001 issue of *Newsweek*—PhRMA, the trade association of America's pharmaceutical companies. The reason I bring this up, is not because I believe this association is the big bad wolf—on the contrary, they have produced remarkable medicines—but I do believe they missed the mark entirely on the subject of hormone replacement. They made broad sweeping claims that our hormones, which were at their peaks when we were most healthy, are actually bad for us, citing two studies that either showed mentally handicapped men, who were castrated, living longer than control subjects (not a very humane study) or women who were not fertile sharing the same fate of longevity. Yet, they failed to remark on women's susceptibility to heart disease and osteoporosis after menopause, when their hormones suddenly take a plunge. They didn't remark on how men after fifty gain visceral fat and lose muscle, both leading them down the road to heart disease. They overlooked the landmark studies that prove through meta-analysis, or doubleblind, placebo-controlled trials that testosterone, estrogen, progesterone, thyroid, and human growth hormone naturally create an environment for "living longer and living better." Do the above studies make sense in light of biological facts that show, when we are young, when our hormones are peaking, we are also at our peak? I emphatically, with study after study to back me up, state no, they do not. It's rare, if farfetched, that you will find people in their twenties or thirties suffering from heart disease, cancer, osteoporosis, or Alzheimer's disease. Why? Because they are *age-related* and independent of hormones, meaning, many times they manifest in the absence or the decline of our hormones.

I've included at the end of this book a simple guide citing important studies and their principal points from prestigious medical journals, validating the use of natural hormone replacement. I did this for two reasons: one, so that you feel secure in your choice for longevity, and two, your doctor will see that what has seemed an improbability in his medical studies for years, is a very real possibility. With this book you can approach your doctor in the lingo he or she understands.

I wrote this book in hopes that both doctors and patients would recognize there is a choice in how we age. Science has revealed and reported in a slew of studies that with optimal supplementation of hormones in women *and* men, we can remain healthy, happy, and prosperous as late into life as possible. The resigned attitude toward aging reflected by science and medical-minded institutions in the past is turning to one of hope and anticipation. Unfortunately this new paradigm of medicine, although contagious, is slow in the catching. This book, therefore, is a catalyst, a starting point, and a tool to inspire you to share with your doctor the need for an all-inclusive approach to medicine. Instead of waiting to treat an age-related illness when it rises, patients and doctors alike should think ahead and consider its prevention rather than its plausibility. We live in a time when great leaps are being made, where science is delving into the improbable realm of genetic splicing and modification. This kind of science is not a viable alternative, yet, presently, as I have enumerated throughout this book, we have the ability to get a handle on how we age—we have a choice and I believe the medium to implement that choice is natural hormone replacement therapy.

Pharmacies of the Past, Reshaping the Future

You should also understand, since I didn't stress this in any of the chapters, that these types of hormones are not found at most general pharmacies. Pharmacies that you find at your local grocery store serve generalities, not particulars. They serve a purpose of convenience and most of your normal pharmaceutical needs—antibiotics, pain medication, or common cold cures. But, natural hormone replacement therapy depends on an entirely precise kind of mixture, and big pharmaceutical companies cannot afford to worry about titration of hormone levels and matching medications to create an optimal therapy for each individual person. Pharmaceutical companies also cannot patent natural hormones without molecularly altering their structure, and this is where side effects come into the picture. Because you are unique, what your body needs or how your body will react to certain doses of a particular hormone is also unique. Therefore, it is important to find a compounding pharmacy with the capabilities of making a hormone to match the *slightest* hormonal variances of your body with the identical hormones your body normally produces.

So, first things first, find a doctor and program that suits your personal health needs. To do this, I suggest you find one that will listen to your symptoms, gauge your personal health goals, and create with you a partnership in longevity. Second, find a pharmacy you can trust. There are several compounding pharmacies in America who specialize in creating bio identical hormones, and who can formulate the exact dosage your doctor believes is right for your body. I, along with many of my colleagues, choose MedQuest Pharmacy for its friendly customer service and high quality standards. I want you to make no mistake, or simply to settle in your pursuit for healthy aging.

Are You Ready?

So, the question is, are you ready to regain your youth? Are you ready to assume your future with the knowledge and wisdom your age suggests, without the wrinkles, the weakness, and the ailments your age suggests? A hormone replacement program that is natural and tailored to your exacting needs can give you that kind of aging—that hardly noticeable aging your friends and family members will claim is your successful secret. With the supplementation of thyroid, testosterone, melatonin, pregnenolone, and DHEA, and the addition of estrogen and progesterone if you are female, along with the inclusion of the healing agent, human growth hormone, you can enjoy the promise of healthy aging. The cliché "happiness truly comes from within" is not too far from the truth. With hormones in their optimal ranges, our beauty and energy can resurface, and future possibilities can reawaken. I encourage you to push the aging envelope. Discover the fountain of youth with ingredients your body has understood since its very conception—hormones.

Let this book jog your curiosity. Let this book be the foundation to your rebirth into the next half of your life. The time is now to shake the stereotype of old age, and regain the confidence you've worked hard to possess. Natural hormone replacement therapy holds the key to unraveling the mystery to a longer, better, and more enjoyable future.

Are you ready?

Bibliography

Bibliography for DHEA

Araghi-Niknam M, Zhang Z, Jiang S, Call O, Eskelson CD, Watson RR. Cytokine dysregulation and increased oxidation is prevented by dehydroepiandrosterone in mice infected with murine leukemia retrovirus. Proc Soc Exp Biol Med 1997 Dec;216(3):386-91.

Barrett-Connor E, Khaw KT, Yen SS. A prospective study of dehydroepiandrosterone sulfate, mortality, and cardiovascular disease. N Eng J Med 1986 Dec;315:1519-24.

Bates, G. et al (1995) "DHEA attenuates study induced declines in insulin sensitivity in postmenopausal women" Ann NY Acad Sci 774: 291-93.

Bloch, M. et al (1999) "Dehydroepiandrosterone treatment of midlife dysthymia" Bio Psychiatry 45: 1533-41.

Casson, P. et al (1995) "Replacement of dehydroepiandrosterone enhances T-lymphocyte insulin sensitivity in post menopausal women" Fertil Steril 63: 1027-31.

Casson, P. et al (1993) "Oral dehydroepiandrosterone in physiologic doses modulates immune function in postmenopausal women" Am J. Obstet Gynecol 169: 1536-39

Danenberg HD, Ben-Yehuda A, Zakay-Rones Z, Friedman G. Dehydroepiandrosterone enhances influenza immunization in aged mice. Ann NY Acad Sci 1995 Dec29; 774:297-9.

Daynes RA, Araneo BA, Ershler WB, Maloney C, Li GZ, Ryu SY. Altered regulation of IL-6 production with normal aging. Possible linkage to the age-associated decline in dehydroepiandrosterone and its sulfated derivative. J Immunol 1993 Jun 15;150(12):5219-30.

Diamond, P. et al (1996) "Metabolic effects of 12-month percutaneous dehydroepiandrosterone replacement therapy in postmenopausal women" J Endocrinol 150:S43-S5.

Feldman FA, Johannes CB, Araujo AB, Mohr BA, Longcope C, McKinlay JB. Low dehydroepiandrosterone and ischemic heart disease in middle-aged men: prospective results from the Massachusetts Male Aging Study. Am J Epidemiol, 2001;153(1):79-89.

Hansen PA, Han DH, Nolte LA, Chen H, Holloszy. DHEA protects against visceral obesity and muscle insulin resistance in rats fed a high-fat diet. Am J Physiol 1997 Nov;273(5 Pt 2):R1704-8.

Hennebold JD, Daynes RA. Regulation of macrophage dehydroepiandrosterone sulfate metabolism of inflammatory cytokines. Endocrinology 1994;135:67-75.

Jakubowicz, D. et al (1995) "Effect of dehydroepiandrosterone on cyclic-guanosine monophosphate in age advance men" Ann NY Acad Sci 774:312-15.

Khalil A, Fortin JP, LeHoux JG, Fulop T. Age-related decrease of dehydroepiandrosterone concentrations in low density lipoproteins and its role in the susceptibility of low density lipoproteins to lipid peroxidation. J Lipid Res 2000;41:1552-61.

Khorram O, Vu L, Yen SS. Activation of Immune function by dehydroepiandrosterone (DHEA) in age-advanced men. J Gerontol A Biol Sci Med Sci 1997 Jan; 52(1):M1-7.

Kimonides VG, Spillantini MG, Sofroniew MV, Fawcett JW, Herbert J. Dehydroepiandrosterone antagonizes the neurotoxic effects of corticosterone and translocation of stress-activated protein kinase 3 in hippocampal primary cultures. Neuroscience 1999 Mar;89(2):429-36.

Kurzman ID, Panciera DL, Miller JB, MacEwen EG. The effect of dehydroepiandrosterone combined with a low-fat diet in spontaneously obese dogs: A clinical trial. Obesity Res 1998; 6(1).

Luo S, Labrie C, Belanger A, Labrie F. Effect of dehydroepiandrosterone on bone mass, serum lipids, and dimethylbens(a)anthracene-induced mammary carcinoma in the rat. Endocrinology 1997 Aug;138(8):3387-94.

Morales A. et al (1994) "Effects of replacement dose of dehydroepiandrosterone in men and women of advancing age." J Clin Endocrinol Metab 78: 1360-67.

Orentreich N, Brind JL, Rizer RL, Vogelman JH. Age changes and sex differences in serum dehydroepiandrosterone sulfate concentrations throughout adulthood. J Clin Endocrinol Metab 1984 Sep; 59(3):551-5.

Regelson W, Carol Coleman. The Super Hormone Promise: Nature's Anecdote to Aging. Pocket Books, New York; 1996.

Riley V, Fitzmaurice MA, Regelson W. DHEA and thymus integrity in the mouse. In: The Biological Role of Dehydroepiandrosterone (DHEA). Kalimi M, Regelson W, Eds., New York: Walter de Gruyter, pp. 131-155, 1990.
Scwartz AG, Pashko LL. Cancer prevention with dehydroepiandros-

terone and non-androgenic structural analogues by Scwartz AG, Pashko LL. J Cell Biochem Suppl 1995; 22:210-7.

Shafagoj Y, Opoku J, Qureshi D, Regelson W, Kalimi M. Dehydroepiandrosterone prevents dexamethasone-induced hypertension in rats. Am J Physiol 1992 Aug;263(2 Pt 1):E210-3.

Solerte SB, Fioravanti M, Vignati G, Giustina A, Cravello L, Ferrari E. Dehydroepiandrosterone sulfate enhances natural killer cell cytotoxicity in humans via locally generated immunoreactive insulin-like growth factor I. J Clin Endocrinol Metab 1999 Sep; 84(9):3260-7.

Bibliography for Pregnenolone

Crook TH, Adderly B. The Memory Cure. New York, NY: Simon and Shuster; 1998.

Flood JF, Morley JE, Roberts E. Memory-enhancing effects in male mice of pregnenolone and steroids metabolically derived from it. Proc Natl Acad Sci USA 1992 Mar 1;89(5):1567-71.

Flood JF, Morley JE, Roberts E. Pregnenolone sulfate enhances post-training memory processes when injected in very low doses into limbic system structures: amygfala is by far the most sensitive. Proc Natl Acad Sci USA1995 Nov 7;92(23):10806-10.

Freeman H, Pincus G, Bachrach S, et al. Therapeutic efficacy of delta 5 pregnenolone in rheumatoid arthritis. JAMA 1950; 143:338-44.

George MS, Guidotti A, Rubinow D, et al. CSF neuroactive steroids in affective disorders: pregnenolone, progesterone and DBI. Biol Psychiatry 1994;35(10):775-80.

Guth L, Zhang Z, Roberts E. Key role for pregnenolone in combination therapy that promotes recovery after spinal cord injury. Proc Natl Acad Sci USA 1994 Dec 6;91 (25):12308-12.

McGavack TH, Chevalley J, Weissberg J. The use Delta 5 pregnenolone in various clinical disorders. J Clin Endocrinol 1951;11(6):559-77.

Meziane H, Mathis C, Paul SM, Ungerer A. The neurosteroid pregnenolone sulfate reduces learning deficits induced by scopamine and has promnestic effects in mice performing an appetitive learning task. Neuropharmacology 1996;126(4):323-30.

Pincus G, Hoagland H. Effects of administered pregnenolone on fatiguing psychomotor performance. J Aviat. Med. 1944;15:98-115.
Pincus G, Hoagland H. Effects on industrial production of the administration of delta 5 pregnenolone to factory workers. I. Psychosomatic Med. 1945;7:342-46.

Schumacher M, Akwa Y, Guennoun R, Robert F, Labombarda F, Desarnaud F, Robel P, De Nicola AF, Baulieu EE. Steroid synthesis and metabolism in the nervous system: trophic and protective effects. J Neurocytol 2000 May-June;29(5-6):307-26.

Steiger A, Trachsel L, Guldner J, et al. Neurosteroid pregnenolone induces sleep-EEG changes in man compatible with inverse agonistic GABA-receptor modulation. Brain Res 1993;615:267-74.

Sternberg TH, LeVan P, Wright ET. The hydrating effects of pregnenolone acetate on the human skin. Curr Ther Res 1961; 3(11):469-71.

Bibliography for Melatonin

Bartsch C, Bartsch H, Schmidt A, Ilg S, Bichler KH, Fluchter SH. Melatonin and 6-sulfatoxymelatonin circadian rhythms in serum and urine of primary prostate cancer patients: evidence for reduced pineal activity and relevance of urinary determinations. Clin Chim Acta1992;209:153-167.

Becker-Andre M, et al. Pineal gland hormone melatonin binds and activates and orphan of the nuclear receptor superfamily. J Bio Chem

1994; 269:28531-28534.

Brzezinksi, A. Melatonin in Humans. 1997;336(3):186-195.

Caroleo MC, Doria G, Nistico G. Melatonin restores immunodepression in aged and cyclophosphamide-treated mice. Ann N Y Acad Sci 1994 May 31;719:343-352.

Coon SL, Roseboom PH, Baler R, et al. Pineal serotonin N-acetyltransferase: expression cloning and molecular analysis. Science 1995;270:1681-1683.

Gonzales-Haba MG, Garcia-Maurino S, Calvo JR, Goberna R, Guerrero JM. High-affinity binding of melatonin by human circulating Tlymphocytes (CD4+). FASEB J 1995; 9:1331-1335.

Lesnikov V, Piepaoli W. Pineal cross-transplantation (old-to-young and vice versa) as evidence for an endogenous "aging clock" Ann N Y Acad Sci 1994; 719: 456-460.

Lissoni P, Barni S, Cazzaniga M, et al. Efficacy of the concomitant administration of the pineal hormone melatonin in cancer immunotherapy with low dose IL-2in patients with advanced solid tumors who had progressed on IL-2 alone. Oncology 1994; 51:344-47.

Lissoni P, Meregalli S, Fossati V, et al. A randomized study of low dose subcutaneous interleuken-2 plus melatonin vs. chemotherapy for advanced non-small cell lung cancer. Tumori 1994; 80:464-67.

Lissoni P, Meragalli S, Nosetto L, et al. Increased survival time in brain glioblastomas by a radioneuroendocrine strategy with radiotherapy plus melatonin compared to radiotherapy alone. Oncology 1996;53:43-46.

Maestroni GJ. The immunoneuroendocrine role of melatonin. J Pineal Res 1993 Jan;14(1):1-10.

Maestroni GJM, Conti A. Melatonin and the pineal gland-from basic science to clinical application. Pp. 295-302, Touitou Y, Arendt J, Pevet P (eds), Elsevier Science Publ., 1993.

Maestroni GJM, Conti A, Lissoni P. Colony-stimulating activity and hematopoietic rescue from cancer chemotherapy compounds are induced by melatonin via endegenous interleukin 4. Cancer Res 1994:54:4740-4743.

Molis TM, Spriggs LL, Hill SM. Modulation of estrogen receptor mRNA expression by melatonin in MCF-7 human breast cancer cells. Mol Endocrinol 1994;8:1681-1690.

Ortiz GG, Sanchez-Ruiz Y, Tan DX, Reiter RJ, Benitez-King G, Beas-Zarate C. Melatonin, vitamin E, and estrogen reduce damage induced by kainic acid in the hippocampus: potassium-stimulated GABA release. J Pineal Res 2001 Aug;31(1): 62-7.

Pierpaoli W, Bulian D, Dall'Ara A. Circadian melatonin and young-to-old grafting postpone aging and maintain juvenile conditions of reproductive functions in mice and rats. Exp Gerontology in press; Abstract: Third Int. Symp. of Neurobiology and Neuroendocrinology of Aging, 1996.

Reiter RJ. The role of the neurohormone melatonin as a buffer against macromolecular oxidative damage. Neurochem Int 1995:27:453-460.

Tan DX, Chen LD, Poeggeler B, Manchester LC, Reiter RJ. Melatonin: a potent, endogenous hydroxyl radical scavenger. Endocr J 1993; 1:57-60.

Tan DX, Poeggeler B, Reiter Rj, et al. The pineal hormone melatonin inhibits DNA-adduct formation induced by the chemical carcinogen safrole in vivo. Cancer Lett 1993; 70:65-71.

Wurtman RJ, et al. Physiologic melatonin doses restore sleep efficiency in insomniac older people. ENDO 2000-The Endocrine Society

82nd Annual Meeting; June 21-24, 2000; Toronto, Canada. Abstract #195. Wurtman RJ. Improvement of sleep quality by melatonin. (letter) Lancet, 1995;346:1491.

Bibliography for Estrogen

Bergkvist L, Adami H-O, Persson I, et al. Prognosis after breast cancer diagnosis in women exposed to estrogen and estrogen-progestogen replacement therapy. Am J Epidem 130;221-227, 1989.

Bostick RM, Potter JD, Kushi LH, et al. Sugar, meat, and fat intake, and non-dietary risk factors for colon cancer incidence in Iowa women (United States). Cancer Causes Control 1994;5:38-52.

Brenner DE, Kukull WA, Stergachis A, et al. Postmenopausal estrogen replacement therapy on the risk of Alzheimer's disease: a population-based case control study. Am J Epidemiol 1994;140:262-267.

Bush TL. Long term effect of estrogen use on cardiovascular death in women. Presentation at: American Heart Association; 1991; Orlando, FL.

Colditz GA, et al. A prospective study of reproductive history and exogenous estrogens on the risk of colorectal cancer in women. Epidemiology 1991;2:201-207.

DiSaia PJ, Grosen EA, Kurosaki T, et al. Hormone replacement therapy in breast cancer survivors: a cohort study. Obstetrics Gynecology 147:1495,1996.

Ditkoff EC, Crary WG, Cristo M, Lobo RA. Estrogen improves psychological function in asymptomatic postmenopausal women. Obstet Gynecol 1991; 78:991-5.

Ettinger, B., Genant, H. K., and Cann, C.E. "Long term estrogen replacement therapy prevents bone loss and fractures." Annals of Internal Medicine 1985; 102:319-324.

Furner SE, Davis FG, Nelson RL, et al. A case-control study of large bowel cancer and hormone exposure in women. Cancer Res 1989;49:4936-4940.

Gerhardsson de Verdier M, London S. Reproductive factors, exogenous female hormones, and colorectal cancer by subsite. Cancer Causes Control 1992;3:355-360.

Grodstein F, Martinez ME, Platz EA, et al. Postmenopausal hormone use and risk for colorectal cancer and adenoma. Ann Intern Med 1998;128:705-712.

Grodstein FM, Stampfer MJ, Manson JE, et al. Postmenopausal estrogen and progestin use and the risk of cardiovascular disease. N Engl J Med 1996;335:453-461.

Henderson BE, Paganini-Hill A, Ross RK. Decreased mortality in users of estrogen replacement therapy. Arch Intern Med 1991;151:75-78.

Herbert-Croteau N. A meta-analysis of hormone replacement therapy and colon cancer in women. Cancer Epidemiol Biomarkers Prev 1998;7:653-659.

Holland, Cecilia. Hot Flashes: Women Writers on the Change of Life. Ed. Lynne Taetzsch. Boston: Faber and Faber, 1995. 26.

Jacobs EJ, White E, Weiss NS. Exogenous hormones, reproductive history, and colon cancer (Seattle, Washington, USA). Cancer Causes Control 1994;5:359-366.

Kampman E, Potter JD, Slattery ML, et al. Hormone replacement therapy, reproductive history, and colon cancer: a multicenter, case-control study in the United States. Cancer Causes Control 1997;8:146-158.

Kawas C, Resnick S, Morrison A, et al. A prospective study of estrogen replacement therapy and the risk of developing Alzheimer's disease: The Baltimore Longitudinal Study of Aging. Neurology

1997;48:1517-1521.

Lando JF, Heck KE, Brett KM. Hormone replacement therapy and breast cancer risk in a nationally representative cohort. Am J Prev Med 1999 Oct; 17(3): 176-80.

Lerner AJ, Koss E, Debanne SM, et al. Interactions of smoking history with estrogen replacement therapy as protective factors for Alzheimer's disease. Presentation at: 26th Annual Meeting of the Society of Neuroscience. 1996; Washington, DC.

Limouzin-Lamothe MA, Mairon N, Joyce CRB, LeGal M. Quality of life after the menopause: influence of hormonal replacement therapy. Am J Obstet Gyn 170:618, 1994.

Morris MS, Jacques PF, Selhub J, Rosenberg IH. Total Homocysteine and estrogen status indicators in the Third National Health and Nutrition Examination Survey. Am J Epidemiol 2000 Jul 15; 152(2);140-8.

Newcomb PA, Storer BE, Marcus PN. Cancer of the large bowel in relation to the use of hormone replacement therapy. Am J Epidemiol 1992;136:958.

Newcomb PA, Storer BE. Postmenopausal hormone use and risk of large-bowel cancer. J Natl Cancer Inst 1995;87:1067-1071.

Newton KM, LaCroix AZ, McKnight B, et al. Estrogen replacement therapy and prognosis after first myocardial infarction. Am J Epidemiol 1997;145:269-277.

Paganini-Hill, A. "The risks and benefits of estrogen replacement therapy: Leisure World." Journal of Fertility and Menopausal Studies 1995:40 (Supp. 1): 54-62.
Paganini-Hill A, Henderson VW. Estrogen replacement therapy and risk of Alzheimer's disease. Arch Intern Med 1996;156:2213-2217.
Risch HA, Howe GR. Menopausal hormone use and colorectal can-

cer in Saskatchewan: a record linkage cohort study. Cancer Epidemiol Biomark Prev 1995;4:21-28.

Rodriguez C, Calle EE, Patel AV, Tatham LM, Jacobs EJ, Thun MJ. Effect of body mass on the association between estrogen replacement therapy and mortality among elderly US women. Am J Epidemiol 2001 Jan 15; 153(2):145-152.

Sauerbronn AV, Fonseca AM, Bagnoli VR, Saldiva PH, Pinotti JA. The effects of systemic hormonal replacement therapy on the skin of postmenopausal women. Int J Gynaecol Obstet 2000 Jan; 68(1):35-41.

Sherwin, B.B. "Sex Hormones and Psychological Functioning in Postmenopausal Women," Exp. Gerontol. 29:423-30,1994.

Stadel BV, Rubin GL, Webster LA, Schlesselman JJ, Wingo PA. Oral contraceptives and breast cancer in young women. Lancet 1985 Nov 2;2(8462):970-3.

Tang M-X, Jacobs D, Stern Y, et al. Effect of oestrogen during menopause on risk and age at onset of Alzheimer's disease. Lancet 1996;348:429-432.

Troisi R, Schairer C, Chow W-H, et al. A prospective study of menopausal hormones and risk of colorectal cancer (United States). Cancer Causes Control 1997;8:130-138.

Wingo PA, Layde PM, Lee NC, Rubin G, Ory Hw. The risk of breast cancer in postmenopausal women who have used estrogen replacement therapy. JAMA 1987 Jan 9;257(2);209-15.

Wolf PH, Madans JH, Finucane FF, et al. Reduction of cardiovascular disease-related mortality among postmenopausal women who use hormones: evidence from a national cohort. Am J Obstet Gynecol 1991;164:489-494.

The Writing Group for the PEPI Trial. Effects of estrogen or estrogen/progestin regimens on heart disease risk factors in postmenopausal women. JAMA 1995;273:199-208.

Bibliography for Progesterone

Adler T. Science News. 1994; 146[22]: 357. Annual scientific meeting of the American Heart Association in Dallas, November 1994.

Carlson CL, Cushman M, Enright PL, Cauley JA, Newman AB. Hormone replacement therapy is associated with higher FEV1in elderly women. Am J Respir Crit Care Med 2001 Feb;163(2):143-8.

Eriksen EF, Langdahl B, Vesterby A, Rungby J, Kassem M. Hormone replacement therapy prevents osteoclastic hyperactivity: A histomorphometric study in early postmenopausal women. J Bone Miner Res 1999; 14(7):1217-21.

Fitzpatrick LA, Pace C, Wiita B. Comparison of regimens containing oral micronized progesterone or medroxyprogesterone acetate on quality of life in postmenopausal women: a cross-sectional survey. J Womens Health Gend Based Med 2000 May; 9.

Giuliani A, Concin H, Wieser F, Boritsch J, Wilfert H, Gruber D, Urdl. Hormone replacement therapy with a transdermal estradiol gel and oral micronized progesterone. Effect on menopausal symptoms and lipid metabolism. Wien Klin Wochenschr 2000 Jul 28;112(14):629-33.

Hargrove JT, Maxson WS, Wentz AC, and Burnett LS. Menopausal hormone replacement therapy with continuous daily oral micronized estradiol and progesterone. Obstetrics & Gynecology 1989; 71,606-612.

Hofseth LJ, Raafat AM, Osuch JR, Pathak DR, Slomski CA, Haslam SZ. Hormone replacement therapy with estrogen or estrogen plus medroxyprogesterone acetate is associated with increased epithelial proliferation in the normal postmenopausal breast. J Clin Endocrinol Metab 1999 Dec; 84 (12): 4559-65.

Lee, J.R. "Osteoporosis Reversal: The Role of Progesterone," Int. Clin. Nutr. Rev. 10:384-91, 1990.

Miller BE, DeSouza MJ, Slade K, Luciano AA. Sublingual administration of micronized estradiol and progesterone, with and without micronized testosterone: effect on biochemical markers of bone metabolism and bone mineral density. Menopause 2000;7:318-326.

Miyagawa K, Rssch J, Stanczyk F, Hermsmeyer K. Medroxyprogesterone interferes with ovarian steroid protection against coronary vasospasm. Nature Med. 1997;3:324-327.

Montplaisir J, Lorrain J, Denesle R, Petit, D. Sleep in menopause: differential effects of two forms of hormone replacement therapy. Menopause 2001; 8:10-16.

Rosano GM, Webb CM, Chierchia S, Morgani GL, Gabraele M, Sarre PM, De Ziegler D, Collins P. Natural progesterone, but not medroxyprogesterone acetate, enhances the beneficial effect of estrogen on exercise-induced myocardial ischemia in postmenopausal women. J Am Coll Cardiol 2000 Dec ;36(7):2154-9.

Ross RK, Paganini-Hill A, Wan PC, Pike MC. Effect of hormone replacement therapy on breast and cancer risk: Estrogen versus estrogen plus progestin. J Natl Cancer Inst 2000;16;92(4):328-32.

Schairer C, Lubin J, Troisi R, et al. Menopausal estrogen-progestin replacement therapy and breast cancer risks. JAMA 2000; 283(4):485-91.

Suriano KA, McHale M, McLaren CE, Li K, Re A, DiSaia PJ. Estrogen replacement therapy in endometrial cancer patients: a matched controlled study. Obstet Gynecol 2001 Apr; 97(4):555-560. Williams JK, Adams MR. Estrogens, progestins, and coronary artery reactivity. Nature Med. 1997;3:273-274.

Bibliography for Testosterone

Aver S., Dobs AS, Meikle AW, et al. Improvement of sexual function in testosterone deficient men treated for one year with a permeation enhanced testosterone transdermal system. J Urol 1996; 155: 1604-8.

Basaria S. Dobs AS. Risks versus benefits of testosterone therapy in elderly men. Drugs Aging 1999; 15 (2): 131-42.

Carter H.B. et al., Longitudinal evaluation of serum androgen levels in men with and without prostate cancer, The Prostate, 1995; 27:25-31.

Davis SR, McCloud P, Strauss BH, Burger H. Testosterone enhances estradiol's effects on postmenopausal bone density and sexuality. Maturitas 1995; 21:227-236.

Gann, P.H., et al., A prospective study of plasma hormone levels, non-hormonal factors, and development of benign prostatic hyperplasia, The Prostate, 1995; 26: 40-49.

Gouras GK, Xu H, Gross RS, Greenfield JP, Hai B, Wang R, Greengard P., Testosterone decreases neuronal secretion of Alzheimer's beta-amyloid peptides. Proc Natl Acad Sci USA 2000 Feb 1;97 (3): 1202-5.

Gulberg B, Johnell O, Kanis JA. World-wide projections for hip fracture. Osteoporosis Int. 1997; 7: 407-413.

Janowsky JS, Chavez B, Orwoll E., Sex steroids modify working memory. J Cogn Neurosci 2000 May; 12(3): 407-14.

Jassal SK, Barrett-Connor E, Edelstein SL. Low bioavailable testosterone levels predict future height loss in postmenopausal women. Journal of Bone Mineral Research. 1995; 10:650-654.

Fran Kaiser, "Testosterone Therapy Shows Promise in Elderly Men,"

Journal of American Geriatrics Society, February 18, 1993.

Katznelson L, Finkelson JS, Schoenfeld DA, et al. Increase in bone density and lean body mass during testosterone administration in men with acquired hypogonadism. J Clin Endocrinol Metab 1996; 81: 4358-65.

Longcope C, Baker RS, Hui SL, Johnston CC Jr. Androgen and estrogen dynamics in women with vertebral crush. Maturitas 1984; 6:309-318.

Manolagas SC. Birth and death of bone cells: basic regulatory mechanisms and implications for the pathogenesis and treatment of osteoporosis. Endocr Rev. 2000; 21:115-137.

Monath, J.R. et al., Physiologic variations of serum testosterone with the normal range do not affect serum prostate specific antigen, Urology, 1995; 46(1):58-61.

Morales A, Johnston B, Heaton JPW, et al. Testosterone supplementation for hypogonadal impotence: assessment of biochemical measures and therapeutic outcomes. J Urol 1997; 157: 849-54.

Oppenheim D, Klibanski A. Osteopenia in men with acquired hypogonadism: improvement with testosterone replacement (Abstract no. 585). Programs and Abstracts of the 71st Meeting of the Endocrine Society; 1989 Jun: 289.

Poggi, UL; et al. Plasma testosterone and serum lipids in male survivors of myocardial infarction, Journal of Steroid Biochemistry, 1976; 7: 229-231.

Raisz L, Wiita B, Arthis A, et al. Comparison of the effects of estrogen alone and estrogen plus androgen on biochemical markers of bone formation and resorption in postmenopausal women. J Clin Endo Metab. 1996; 81:37-43.

Robert J. Paradowski, The American Academic Encyclopedia (1995 Grolier Multimedia Encyclopedia Version) on CD-Rom Copyright 1995 Grolier, Inc., Danbury Conn.

Reported in Third Age Media, Thirdagemedia.com, 13 March, 1999.

Sarrel P, Dobay, Wiita B. Estrogen and estrogen-androgen replacement in postmenopausal women dissatisfied with estrogen-only therapy. Sexual behavior and neuroendocrine responses. J Reprod Med 1998 Oct;43(10)847-56.

Schatzl G, Madersbacher S, Thurridl T, Waldmuller J, Kramer G, Haitel A, Marberger M. High-grade prostate cancer is associated with low serum testosterone levels. Prostate 2001 Apr; 47(1):52-8.

Shalender Bhasin et al., "The Effects of Suprahysiologic Doses of Testosterone on Muscle Size and Strength in Normal Men," New England Journal of Medicine 335, no. 1 (July4, 1996):1-7.

Shapiro J, Christiana J, Frishman WH. Testosterone and other anabolic steroids as cardiovascular drugs. Am J Ther 1999 May; 6(3):167-74.

Sherwin B.B., (1988) Affective changes with estrogen and androgen replacement therapy in surgically menopausal women. J Affect. Disord. 14, 177-187.

Shrifen J, Braunstein G, Siman J, et al. Transdermal testosterone treatment in women with impaired sexual function and psychological well-being in oophorectomized women. N Engl. J Med. 2000; 343:682-688.

Sih R, Morley JE , Kaiser FE, et al. Testosterone replacement in older hypogonadal men: a 12-month randomized controlled trial. J Clin Endocrinol Metab 1997: 82: 1661-7.

Slater S, Oliver RT. Testosterone: its role in development of prostate cancer and potential risk from use as hormone replacement therapy. Drugs Aging 2000 Dec;17(6):431-9.

Suzuki, K., et al., Endocrine environment of benign prostatic hyperplasia: prostate size and volume are correlated with serum estrogen concentration, Scandinavian Journal of Urology and Nephrology, 1995; 29: 65-68.

United States Dept. of Statistics of the United States, National Center for Health Statistics, Vital Statistics of the United States, Table 8-5.

Vermeulen A, Kaulman JM. "Aging of the Hypothalmo-Pituitary Testicular Axis in Men," Hormonal Research 43, no. 1-3 (1995): 25-28.

Wang C., Eyre DR, Clark R, et al. Sublingual testosterone replacement improves muscle mass and strength, decreases bone resorption, and increases bone formation markers in hypogonadal men: a clinical research center study. J Clin Endocrinol Metab1996; 81: 3654-62.

Waxenberg, S. E., M. G. Drellich, A. M. Sutherland, The role of hormones in Human Behavior. I. Changes in female sexuality after adrenalalectomy. J Clin Endo 19 (1959)193-202.

Webb CM, McNeill JG, Hayward CS, de Ziegler D, Collins P. Effects of testosterone on coronary vasomotor regulation in men with coronary heart disease. Circulation 1999 Oct 19; 100(16): 1690-6.

Wehren LE, Hawkes W, Zimmerman SI, et al. Mortality among men after hip fracture (abstract). J Bone Miner Res. 2000; 15(suppl 1) :S223.

Zgliczynski S; et al., Effect of testosterone replacement therapy on lipids and lipoproteins in hypogonadal and elderly men. Atherosclerosis 1996 Mar; 121(1):35-43.

Bibliography for Thyroid

Barnes, B.O. and L. Galton, Hypothyroidism: The Unsuspected Illness. New York: Harper and Row, 1976.

Barnes, B. Basal temperature verses basal metabolism, J Am Med Assoc. 119 (1942): 1072-74.

Bengel FM, Nekolla SG, Ibrahim T, Weniger C, Ziegler S, Schwaiger M. Effect of thyroid hormones on cardiac function, geometry, and oxidative metabolism assessed noninvasively by position emission tomography and magnetic resonance imaging. J Clin Endocrinol Metab 2000;85:1822-7.

Bunevicius R, Kazanavicius G, Zalinkevicius R, Prange AJ Jr. Effects of thyroxine as compared with thyroxine plus triiodothyronine in patients with hypothyroidism. N Engl J Med. 1999 Feb 11;340(6):424-9.

Crowley WF Jr, Ridgeway EC, Bough EW, et al. Noninvasive evaluation of cardiac function in hypothyroidism: response to gradual thyroxine replacement. N Engl J Med 1997296:1-6.

Danese MD, Powe NR, Sawin CT, Ladenson PW. Screening for mild thyroid failure in the periodic health examination: a decision and cost-effective analysis. JAMA 1996:276:285-92.

Escobar-Morreale HF, del Ray FE, Obregon MJ, de Escobar GM. Only the combined treatment with thyroxine and triiodothyronine ensures euthyroidism in all tissues of the thyroidectomized rat. Endocrinology 1996;137:2490-502.

Franklyn JA, Gammage MD, Ramsden DB, Sheppard MC. Thyroid status in patients after acute myocardial infarction. Clin Sci (Colch) 1984;67:585-90.

Gerald S. Levey. Hypothyroidism: A Treacherous Masquerader. Acute Care Medicine May, 1984, pgs 34-36.

Hak AE, Pols HAP, Visser TJ, et al. Subclinical hypothyroidism is an independent risk factor for atherosclerosis and myocardial infarction in elderly women: the Rotterdam Study. Ann Intern Med. 2000;

132:270-78.

Hamilton MA, Stevenson LW, Fonarow GC, et al. Safety and hemodynamic effects of intravenous triiodothyronine in advanced congestive heart failure. Am J Cardiol 1998;81:443-7.

Hoskins, Roy G., The Biology of Schizophrenia. New York: W.W. Norton & Co., Inc., 1946, 110.

Hussein WI, Green R, Jacobsen DW, Faiman C. Normalization of hyperhomocysteinemia with L-thyroxine in hypothyroidism. Ann Intern Med 1999 Sep 7;131(5):348-51.

Klein I, Ojamaa K. The cardiovascular system in hypothyroidism. In: Braverman LE, Utiger RD, eds. Werner & Ingbar's the thyroid: a fundamental and clinical text. 8th ed. Philadelphia: Lippincott Williams & Wilkins, 2000:777-82.

Klemperer JD, Klein I, Gomez M, et al. Thyroid hormone treatment after coronary-artery bypass surgery. N Engl J Med 1995; 333:1522-7.

Ladenson PW, Singer PA. Ain KB, Bagchi N, Bigos ST, Levy EG, Smith SA, Daniels GH. American Thyroid Association guidelines for detection of thyroid dysfunction. Arch Intern Med 2000 Jun 12; 160(11):1573-5.

Ladenson PW, Sherman SI, Baughman RL, Ray PE, Feldman, AM. Reversible alterations in myocardial gene expression in a young man with dilated cardiomyopathy and hypothyroidism. Proc Natl Acad Sci USA 1992;89:5251-5.

Moruzzi P, Doria E, Agostoni PG, Medium-term effectiveness of L-thyroxine treatment in idiopathic dilated cardiomyopathy. Am J Med 1996;101:461-7.

Park KW, Dai HB, Ojamaa K, Lowenstein E, Klein I, Sellke FW. The direct vasomotor effect of thyroid hormones on rat skeletal muscle resistance arteries. Anesth Analg 1997;85:734-8.

Shoman, Mary, "Survey: What Are the Worst Symptoms if Thyroid Disease? Patients Speak Out About Their Key Thyroid Symptoms." About.com Guide to Thyroid Disease.

Thyroid Hormones: Positive Relationships with Cognition in Healthy Euthyroid Older Men. J Gerontol: Medical Science 1999; 54A(3):M111-M116.

Thyroid Society: http://houston-interweb.com/thyroid/faq/33.html

Wren, J. C. Thyroid function and coronary atherosclerosis. J Am Geriatr Soc. 1968 Jun;16(6):696-704.

Bibliography for HGH

Baum HB, Biller BM, Finkelstein JS, Cannistraro KB, Oppenhein DS, Schoenfeld DA, Michel TH, Wittink H, Klibanski A. Effects of physiologic growth hormone therapy on bone density and body composition in patients with adult-onset growth hormone deficiency. A randomized, placebo-controlled trial. Ann Intern Med 1996 Dec 1;125(11):932-4.

Bengtsson BA, Kippeschaar HPF, Abs R, Monson JP, Feldt-Rasmussen U, Wuster, Christian. Letters to the Editor. Growth hormone replacement therapy is not associated with any increase in mortality. J Clin Endocrin Metab 1999;84(11):4291-4292.

Black MM, Shuster s, Bottoms E. Skin Collagen and thickness in acromegaly and hypopituitarism. Clin Endocrinol (Oxf.) 1972;1:259-263.

Bocchi EA, Massuda Z, Guilherme G, Carrara D, Bellotti G, Mecelin A, Rodriguez Sobrinho CR, Ramires JF. Growth hormone for optimization of refractory heart failure treatment. Arq Bras Cardiol 1999 Oct; 73(4):391-8.

Carroll, PV, Littlewood R, Weissberger AJ, Bogalho P, McGauley G, Sonksen PH, Russell-Jones DL. The effects of two doses of replacement growth hormone on the biochemical, body composition, and psychological profiles of growth hormone-deficient adults. Eur J Endocrinol 1997 Aug;137(2):146-53.

Cittadini A, Grossman JD, Napoli R, et al. Growth hormone attenuates early left ventricular remodeling and improves cardiac function in rats with large myocardial infarction. J Am Coll Cardiol 1997;29:1109-16.

Cowell CT, Wuster C. The effects of growth hormone deficiency and growth hormone replacement therapy on bone. A meeting report. Horm Res 2000;54 Suppl 1:68-74.

Christ ER, Carroll PV, Russell-Jones DL, Sonksen PH. The consequences of growth hormone deficiency in adulthood, and the effects of growth hormone replacement. Schweiz Med Wochenschr 1997 Aug 30;127(35):1440-9.

Cummings MH, Christ E, Umpleby AM, Albany E, Wierzbicki A, Lumb PJ, Sonksen PH, Russell-Jones DL. Abnormalities of very low-density lipoprotein apolipoprotein B-100 metabolism contribute to the dyslipidaemia of adult growth hormone deficiency. J Clin Endocrinol Metab 1997 Jun;82(6):2010-3.

Fazio S, Sabatini D, Capaldo B, Vigorito C, Giordano A, Guida R, Pardo F, Biondi B, Sacca L. A preliminary study of growth hormone in the treatment of dilated cardiomyopathy. N Engl J Med 1996 Mar 28;334(13):809-14.

Genth-Zotz S, Zotz R, Geil S, Voigtlander T, Meyer J, Darius H. Recombinant growth hormone therapy in patients with ischemic cardiomyopathy. Circulation 1999;99:18-21.

Giusti M, Meineri I, Malagamba D, Cuttica CM, Fattacciu G, Menichini U, Rasore E, Giordan G. Impact of recombinant human growth hormone treatment on psychological profiles in hypopituitary patients with adult-onset growth hormone deficiency. Eur J Clin Invest 1998 Jan;28(1):13-9.

Goeddel DV, Heyneker HL, Hozumi T, et al. Direct expression in Escherichia coli of DNA sequence coding for human growth hormone. Nature 1979; 281:544-8.

Kim KR, Nam SY, Song YD, Lim SK, Lee HC, Huh KB. Low-dose growth hormone treatment with diet restriction accelerates body fat loss, exerts anabolic effect and improves growth hormone secretory dysfunction in obese adults. Horm Res 1999;511(2):78-84.

Kotler DP, Wang J, Pierson RN. Body composition studies in patients with the acquired immunodeficiency syndrome. Am J Clin Nutr 1985;42:1255-1265.

Krentz AJ, Koster FT, Crist DM, et al. Anthropometric, metabolic, and immunological effects of recombinant human growth hormone in AIDS and AIDS-related complex. J Acquir Immune Defic Syndr 1993;6:245-251.

Lange KH, Isaksson F, Juul A, Rasmussen MH, Bulow J, Kjaer M. Growth hormone enhances effects of endurance training on oxidative muscle metabolism in elderly women. Am J Physiol Endocrinol Metab 2000 Nov; 279(5):989-96.
Lombardi G, Di Somma C, Marzulla P, Cerbone G, Colao A. Growth hormone and cardiac function. Ann Endocrinol (Paris) 2000 Feb; 61(1):16-21.

Raben MS. Treatment of a pituitary dwarf with human growth hormone. J Clin Endocrinol Metab 1958; 18:301-3.
Rosen T, Bengtsson BA. Premature mortality due to cardiovascular disease in hypopituitarism. Lancet 1990 Aug 4;336(8710):285-8.

Rosen T, Wiren L, Wilhelmsen L, Wiklund I, Bengtsson BA. Decreased psychological well-being in adult patients with growth hormone deficiency. Clin Endocrinol (Oxf.) 1994;40:111-116.

Rudman D, Feller AG, Nagraj HS, Gergans GA, Lalitha PY, Goldberg AF, Schlenker RA, Cohn L, Rudman IW, Mattson DE. Effects of human growth hormone in men over 60 years old. N Eng J Med 1990 Jul, 323 (1):1-6.

Schambelan M, Mulligan K, Grunfeld C, et al. Recombinant human growth hormone in patients with HIV-associated wasting: a randomized, placebo-controlled trial. Ann Intern Med 1996;125:873-882.
Takala J, Ruokonen E, Webster NR, et al. Increased mortality associated with growth hormone treatment in critical ill adults. N Engl J Med 1999;341:785-792.

Vance ML, Mauras N. Growth Hormone Therapy in Adults and Children. N Eng J Med 1999;341(16):1206-14.

Verhelst J, Abs R, Vandewdeghe M, Mockel J, Legros JJ, Copinschi G, Mahler C, Velkeniers B, Vanhaelst L, Van Aelst A, De Rijdt D, Stevenaert A, Beckers A. Two years of replacement therapy in adults with growth hormone deficiency. Clin Endocrinol (Oxf) 1997 Oct;47(4):485-94.

Wuster C, Abs R, Bengtsson BA, Bennmarker H, Feldt-Rasmussen U, Hernberg-Stahl E, Monson JP, Westberg B, Wilton P; The KIMS Study Group and the KIMS International Board. Pharmacia & Upjohn International Metabolic Database. The influence of growth hormone deficiency, growth hormone replacement therapy, and other aspects of hypopituitarism on fracture rate and bone mineral density...J Bone Miner Res 2001 Feb;16(2):398-405.

Yang R, Bunting S, Gillet N, Clark R, Jin H. Growth hormone improve cardiac performance in experimental heart failure. Circulation 1995;92(2):262-7.

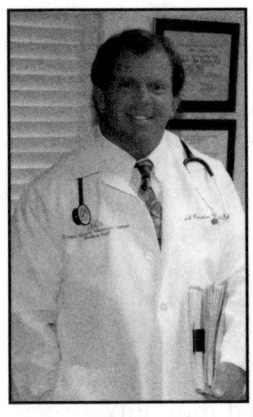

Dr. Neal Rouzier is an innovator and leader in the research, development, and art of longevity medicine. The Preventive Medicine Clinics of the Desert specialize in the evaluation and treatment of hormonal and nutritional deficiencies. The key features of the clinics include individualized treatment programs, continued monitoring, updated therapy, and specialized service that allow for unlimited personal contact with the physician to meet specific needs.

Dr. Rouzier also lectures on the radio and TV and is a frequent speaker for professional medical associations.

2825 Tahquitz Canyon Blvd. Suite 200
Palm Springs, CA. 92662
Ph: (760)320-4292
Fax: (760)322-9475

77564B Country Club Drive, Suite 320
Palm Desert, CA. 92211
Ph: (760) 772-8883
Fax: (760)772-8663
www.hormonedoctor.com
hormonedoc@earthlink.net

Cherie Constance is a writer/researcher at MedQuest Pharmacy. Extremely well versed in the field of longevity medicine, she brings a unique perspective to the potential surrounding hormone replacement therapy.
cconstance@mqrx.com

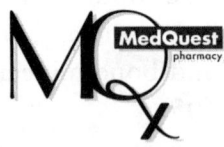

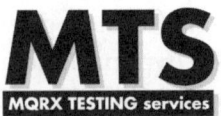

MEDQUEST PHARMACY
6965 Union Park Center, Suite 100
Midvale, Utah 84047
Ph: (888) 222-2956
Fax: (801) 569-0462
info@mqrx.com

MEDQUEST TESTING SERVICE
HORMONE TESTING PANELS
Ph: (888) 556.5567
Fax: (801) 255-7832

www.mqrx.com